SECOND EDITION

WHY PATIENTS SUE DOCTORS

LESSONS LEARNED FROM MEDICAL MALPRACTICE CASES

DUNCAN GRAHAM

BERNARD KELLY

DAVID RICHARDS

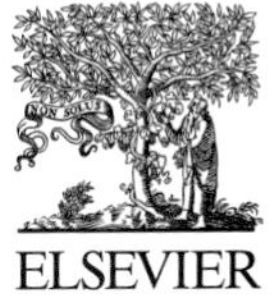

ELSEVIER

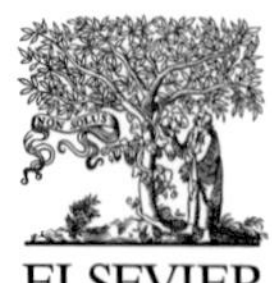

Elsevier Australia. ACN 001 002 357
(a division of Reed International Books Australia Pty Ltd)
Tower 1, 475 Victoria Avenue, Chatswood, NSW 2067

ISBN: 978-0-7295-4370-5

Notice

Practitioners and researchers must always rely on their own experience and knowledge in evaluating and using any information, methods, compounds or experiments described herein. Because of rapid advances in the medical sciences, in particular, independent verification of diagnoses and drug dosages should be made. To the fullest extent of the law, no responsibility is assumed by Elsevier, authors, editors or contributors for any injury and/or damage to persons or property as a matter of products liability, negligence or otherwise, or from any use or operation of any methods, products, instructions, or ideas contained in the material herein.

National Library of Australia Cataloguing-in-Publication Data

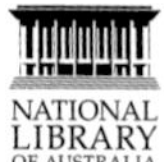

A catalogue record for this book is available from the National Library of Australia

Content Strategist: Larissa Norrie
Content Project Manager: Shruti Raj
Edited by Tim Learner
Cover by Alice Weston
Index by Innodata Indexing
Typeset by Toppan Best-set Premedia Limited
Printed in China by RR Donnelley

Last digit is the print number: 9 8 7 6 5 4 3 2 1

AUTHORS

Duncan Graham SC, MBBS, LLB (Hons), FACLM
Duncan Graham is a barrister with a medical degree. He previously worked as a medical practitioner and solicitor. He now specialises in medical negligence, coronial inquests, professional misconduct and class actions involving pharmaceuticals and medical devices.

Bernard Kelly AM, BSc (Med) (Hons), MBBS, FRACGP
Bernard Kelly is a general practitioner who works in metropolitan, rural and remote locations. He has extensive experience in teaching and medical regulation. He provides expert witness opinions in medical negligence and professional misconduct cases.

David Richards OAM, BSc (Med) (Hons), MBBS, MD, FRACP
David Richards is a physician, with broad experience in clinical and interventional cardiology, education and research. He provides expert witness opinions for plaintiffs, defendants and government agencies.

FOREWORD TO SECOND EDITION

In the old days they used to call it Medical Jurisprudence. Teaching the basics of medical law to medical students.

There are two things that I recall from those lectures during a cold winter in North Eastern Scotland. One has absolutely no relevance to this book but I'll tell you anyway. For some reason, bestiality came up. I was perplexed and couldn't see for the life of me why it was in a Medical Jurisprudence course. I put up my hand from the back of the lecture theatre and asked in a loud voice: "Is bestiality really a crime?" A hard one to live down, and was enshrined in the Final Year Book as my quote.

The second thing I recall was the wise person at the front telling us, emphatically, that we will never be sued by a patient who likes and respects us. Loaded words, and I don't know if it applies today but perhaps finds echoes in Open Disclosure which is about empathy, mutual respect and honesty.

Patients tend to assume that as doctors, we're technically competent. All too often where we falter is in our non-technical skills. The case studies in this book illustrate that ignorance is not often the cause of the errors which lead to litigation. The causes are poor relationships, not listening to what the patient and her family is really telling us, not realising there is a mismatch of expectations, not having systems in place which lower the risk of error and so on.

Information asymmetry is rife in health care and makes it dangerous and inefficient. Usually information asymmetry is expressed as the health care provider knowing more than the patient and family. That gives rise to the most frustrating litigation of all: allegations of failure to inform. But in the case of most litigation, I suspect for once in health care the asymmetry is the other way around. The patient and the people around him often know far more about the problem and its impact and perhaps even its causes than the doctor.

We come to consultations with preconceived ideas; we jump to conclusions based on inadequate information, and we allow prejudice to affect our judgment at our peril, but most importantly of all, at the patient's peril.

Now in its second edition, this book presents more cases to ponder and learn from, including cases from disciplinary proceedings. It can help all of us to avoid the errors in care that lead to litigation. This book can help everyone to avoid the errors in care that lead to litigation.

Norman Swan
Host, *The Health Report*
ABC Radio National

ACKNOWLEDGEMENTS

We acknowledge all those who have enabled us to write the second edition of this book. The list starts with the patients and doctors we have encountered, and continues with the lawyers and government agencies that have referred matters to us over several decades, and sought our opinions.

We have discussed many of the matters in the course of professional review and education, and appreciate the feedback we have received. The clinical lessons we have identified have been refined by the conversations we have had with students, doctors and others.

We thank everyone who has provided feedback from the first edition and reviewed this second edition. The final result is our synthesis, from a plethora of medicolegal cases, of some essential lessons to improve clinical care. Any errors or deficiencies in the text are ours.

CONTENTS

INTRODUCTION

Why do patients sue their doctors? The answer to this question is complex. There are many factors at play. While there may be many patient and social factors relevant to the decision to complain about medical treatment, in essence, patients sue their doctors because of their belief that an error has occurred. There can be no medical negligence or professional misconduct without mistakes. The mistake may be about treatment, diagnosis, judgment, insight or ethics. We have been involved in medicolegal cases for three decades. During that time, we have had first-hand experience of the miscellany of reasons for medical negligence or misconduct litigation.

One of us (DG) has conducted medical malpractice cases for almost 25 years. Two of us (BK and DR) have been involved as expert witnesses for more than 30 years. Based on our collective experience, we aim in this book to provide some insights into medicolegal litigation and to identify the reasons why doctors make mistakes. In this way, we will endeavour to answer the question why patients sue their doctors. In addition, we hope to provide practical guidance to improve clinical care, and to avoid litigation in the future. In this second edition we have included additional illustrative cases of doctors sued by patients, and expanded discussion of the reasons why doctors were sued.

Together we have been engaged in more than 1,000 cases, covering a broad range of issues, over many years. Each of us was struck by the similarities of issues in many cases. Several of the cases, with appropriate deidentification of the individuals involved, have been used to teach medical and legal colleagues how clinical action or inaction may lead to litigation. Analysis of these cases has enabled us to identify strategies for doctors to improve clinical care. Now we would like to share this experience with a wider audience.

When patients have been asked why they initiated a complaint, some will answer that they simply sought to discover the truth. Others may sue doctors because they are angry at the conduct of the doctor and the way the mistake was handled. Often, a simple apology would have forestalled litigation.

Other patients sue doctors because they believe that the compensation will have real benefits in alleviating the suffering or disabilities arising from injuries caused by negligent treatment. Some patients are not interested in money but want to ensure that other patients do not have to suffer the consequences of mistreatment by a particular doctor. There may be an element of wanting to punish a doctor for the harm that has been done or the way they have behaved.

All patients who sue their doctors feel aggrieved by the medical treatment they have received. They will have suffered harm, or believe they have suffered harm, as a consequence of medical mistakes.

Medical practitioners are only human and inevitably will make mistakes at some time. Not all mistakes result in litigation. Not all mistakes should lead to litigation. A doctor is not liable to pay damages to a patient for negligence simply because a mistake has occurred. Fault must be established with credible evidence and, in particular, credible expert evidence. It is up to lawyers to distinguish between simple errors, say of clinical judgment, and conduct or omissions amounting to demonstrable negligence. The same applies to regulatory agencies charged with responsibility for the investigation of complaints or prosecution for misconduct.

THE MEDICOLEGAL PROCESS

While this is not a legal textbook, it is nonetheless important to understand the legal framework within which the cases we describe have occurred. This will help explain the role of the lawyer in separating complaints from patients into matters that do and do not have prospects of success, and assist in understanding why most cases settle without the need for a trial.

LAWYERS AND COURTS

Although we describe cases in Australia, the problems of medical practice we highlight are relevant in all countries.

The benchmark against which the conduct of a medical practitioner is measured is reasonableness. This is the case at common law and under the *Civil Liability Act* 2002 (NSW) and cognate legislation throughout the states and territories of Australia. At common law, the standard of care is that of an ordinary skilled medical practitioner (of the type in question) acting reasonably. Under the Liability Acts, the standard of care is that of a reasonable medical practitioner in the position of the practitioner under scrutiny.

The scope of a medical practitioner's duty involves an assessment of what is reasonable in all the circumstances of the case. This largely requires analysis of what steps are considered reasonable to avoid or ameliorate not insignificant risks of harm associated with proposed management.

In each specific case this involves weighing up the consequences to a patient should a risk materialise, against the cost and difficulty of preventing the particular risk. If a medical practitioner failed to exercise reasonable care and skill against a not insignificant risk of harm, then the doctor will be found to have breached his or her duty of care to the patient.

Once breach of duty of care is established, a court must determine whether that breach was a necessary condition of the harm suffered by the patient. This is known as causation. It entails a "but for" enquiry: whether in the absence of the defendant's negligence, harm would have been occasioned to the plaintiff.

A medical practitioner can defend a claim in negligence if he or she can show that his or her conduct was in accordance with a practice widely accepted at the relevant time by peer professional opinion.

The authors have either given or read many opinions on questions about breach of duty of care and causation over the past three decades. Often, causation questions concern counterfactual or hypothetical situations where experts must give evidence about what theoretically would have occurred if a particular medical practitioner had not breached the duty of care to a patient. These hypothetical analyses can be quite complex because they may require an expert to trace through what would have eventuated if the management of a patient had taken two or more different paths. This is one of the reasons medical negligence litigation is commonly believed to be very difficult.

Most medicolegal problems are settled by mediation, with only a few reaching a court hearing. Even so, the simplest problem usually takes several years to resolve, aggravating stress on the parties involved. If the matter proceeds to court, the hearing is usually more than five years after the event. If the patient is an infant the court hearing may be several decades after the event. In the meantime the practitioner, the subject of the complaint, sits Damocles-like, waiting with dread for the hair to snap. The effect of a complaint or litigation on a medical practitioner is varied. We do not canvass the issue in this book. The subject, however, is important, as doctors should be trained about what to expect when they receive a complaint. It is a largely overlooked area of academic discourse.

The fact that a complaint has arisen does not necessarily mean that it has substance, and many complaints are either considered to be trivial or not sufficiently robust to warrant litigation.

A century ago, it was unusual for patients to sue their doctors. Doctors were put on a pedestal and trusted implicitly that they were doing the best for their patients. Through our experience in medicolegal cases, we have seen a steady increase in medical negligence litigation over the last thirty years.

It is unlikely that medical practitioners have become more negligent. Rather, litigation has become more acceptable. Access to legal advice is easier, especially with the advent of "no win, no fee" arrangements with solicitors. Patients demand more of their doctors. They are more likely to hold them accountable for mistakes. The days of patients putting blind faith in doctors are over.

There are many reasons why an injured patient may consult lawyers and seek to sue a medical practitioner. It is a big step for a layperson to consult a lawyer. Many patients have legitimate cause for concern as a result of the treatment they received. Whether they have a claim requires accurate analysis and investigation by their lawyers. This does not always take place. Some law firms set targets for the number of cases that must be filed within a certain period, such as a month. This leads to spurious claims being mounted against medical practitioners with little or no prospect of success. The claims may be based on the opinions of medical experts who are known to assist one party or another, or an opinion based on assumptions that can never be proved.

Having said this, however, the overwhelming majority of claims that are litigated have some merit even if the plaintiff's lawyers have not clearly identified the mistake or its import. Experts have a duty to the court to provide unbiased and objective opinions, irrespective of whether they are engaged by the plaintiff or the defence. The majority of experts take this obligation seriously. Sometimes the court requests a joint report by experts for the plaintiff and the defence; the report identifies points of agreement and disagreement, and reasons for disagreement.

If a matter does proceed to court the experts are obliged to attend and justify their opinions. On some occasions, experts provide evidence concurrently, to allow the court to understand better the sources of disagreement between witnesses. If the matter is settled by mediation without a court hearing, as most are, the experts are not privy to the outcome, as this is confidential between the plaintiff and the defendant.

Compensation and Costs

A patient or a party on behalf of a patient (the plaintiff) sues a doctor only after the plaintiff's legal team takes a statement from the plaintiff, obtains the relevant clinical records, reviews the facts, receives a favourable opinion from an independent expert, and prepares a claim. The legal team may comprise one or more solicitors and paralegals, one or more barristers and one or more expert witnesses. The legal team and the plaintiff discuss costs and agree on methods of payment prior to any work being performed. As the majority of plaintiffs do not have the financial capacity to pay the costs of their legal team or expert reports, the plaintiff and his or her legal team usually agree that legal costs will be paid out of the settlement amount in the event that the plaintiff's claim is successful.

The sued doctor (the defendant) is invariably represented by a medical defence insurer, who engages a legal team (one or more solicitors and paralegals, one or more barristers and one or more expert witnesses) for the defendant. The legal team and the insurer discuss costs and agree on methods of payment before any legal services are provided. The legal team is conventionally paid on an hourly or daily rate as the matter proceeds.

If a matter is settled before trial, the plaintiff receives an amount (confidential) from the defendant's insurer agreed upon by all parties. The settlement is usually inclusive of the plaintiff's legal costs. The net benefit received by the plaintiff may be reduced in part by the costs of the plaintiff's legal team and paybacks to Medicare or Centrelink. The insurer also pays the defendant's legal team.

If a matter goes to trial, additional court costs are incurred. These costs can be significant. If the plaintiff's claim is successful, costs are paid by the defendant's insurer. If the plaintiff's claim is unsuccessful, then the plaintiff and his or her legal team do not receive any payment. The plaintiff will be liable for the defendant's legal costs. The plaintiff often does not have the financial resources to pay the defendant's costs.

Accordingly, the plaintiff is generally keen for an early and fair settlement, and to avoid the increasing financial and psychological costs of a protracted contest. As the plaintiff's legal team is usually paid if the claim is successful, the more protracted the contest, the greater the potential loss to the legal team if the claim proves unsuccessful. Conversely, if the case against the defendant is strong (or liability has been admitted by the defendant), the more protracted the litigation, the greater the potential return in legal fees to the plaintiff's legal team.

As a general rule, the defendant is less bothered financially by the duration of the contest because the hourly costs of the legal team are underwritten by the insurer. The insurer, however, is interested in minimising expense and may prefer an early commercial resolution. In addition, a protracted contest will likely have emotional and professional consequences for the defendant. If the defendant's legal team is paid by the hour, the more protracted the contest, the greater the income to the legal team.

Legal costs is a complex area of the law requiring specialised knowledge. There are strategies available to the parties to minimise the costs of proceedings such as the making of offers of compromise.

Medical Regulatory Bodies

Medical care throughout the world is regulated to a greater or lesser degree. Doctors registered in Australia are accountable to five regulatory bodies: The Australian Health Practitioner Regulatory Agency (AHPRA), The Professional Services Review (PSR), the Medicare Participation Review Committee (MPRC), the Health Care Complaints Commission (HCCC) in New South Wales (and similar bodies in the other states and territories) and the Australian Medical Council (AMC).

AHPRA maintains the register of all health professionals in Australia and, as far as medical practitioners are concerned, receives and acts upon advice from other bodies about the competence and performance of practitioners.

Complaints reach the state branch of the AMC directly from patients or concerned practitioners, or via the HCCC. The AMC maintains a register of medical practitioners (but not all health professionals). Each state Medical Council (previously state Medical Board) has powers to interview, monitor and discipline doctors. It may suspend the registration of a practitioner for various reasons including incompetence, inadequate record keeping, substance abuse and inappropriate interpersonal behaviour towards patients.

The PSR is the Commonwealth body responsible for protecting the public purse in relation to Medicare billing. The MPRC examines those practitioners who have twice been required to attend a hearing of the PSR. The functions of MPRC are to be subsumed into the PSR.

The HCCC receives complaints from various sources, including directly from patients, and cooperates with the AMC in the investigation and management of these complaints. Disputed complaints are litigated before an administrative tribunal. Appeals are heard in state supreme courts.

It may be alleged that a doctor has engaged in unsatisfactory professional conduct or professional misconduct. These expressions are defined in the

Health Practitioner National Law and include conduct significantly below the standard reasonably expected of a practitioner of an equivalent training and experience (unsatisfactory professional conduct) and unsatisfactory professional conduct of a sufficiently serious nature to justify suspension or cancellation of registration. A tribunal must be comfortably satisfied on the balance of probabilities that the complaint has been made out. Various penalties may be imposed, including deregistration.

OUTLINE OF THIS BOOK

All of the examples we describe are based on true medicolegal cases. Pseudonyms for patients and doctors are used throughout. Dates and locations may be changed. The cases are arranged in regional order of medical complaint, from head to toe. Although we are critical of some clinical actions and inactions, we acknowledge that the vast majority of medical encounters do not lead to complaints or litigation. It is our view that by addressing some of the behaviours of doctors that have led to complaints by patients and their families, we may be able to help practitioners in the future avoid some of the common clinical pitfalls of the past. It is axiomatic that people learn from mistakes. The same is true of professionals. Rather than considering that mistakes should be kept quiet, we think that they should be out in the open. They can provide invaluable aids for medical education.

In the next chapter we describe seven situations where doctors have acted outside appropriate boundaries or acted unethically. The other clinical chapters are case presentations selected from five broad categories: general practice including paediatrics, emergency medicine, surgery, obstetrics and medicine including psychiatry. Each case is presented in a similar format: history, legal issues, discussion and clinical principles. Some cases illustrate multiple deficiencies in care, and many of the deficiencies in care occur in multiple cases.

The case presentation chapters are followed by a consideration of several actions and inactions associated with clinical blindspots and roadblocks. The final chapter highlights the lessons learned from the preceding chapters.

We have not endeavoured to deal comprehensively with all medicolegal topics, nor have we covered all clinical specialties. Rather we have focused on broad classes of issues, in order to identify particular areas of practice that might be improved. We are not attempting to make neurosurgeons better at neurosurgery or general practitioners adhere to impossible standards. We hope that the book will assist in making all doctors better doctors by understanding why mistakes are made across multiple disciplines.

ETHICAL ISSUES

This chapter includes seven examples of inappropriate behaviours by doctors.

COGNITIVE IMPAIRMENT

History

Dr Charles Abernethy, a long-term procedural rural practitioner, was approaching his twilight years. His patients gradually sought medical care from other practitioners in the town, such that Dr Abernethy's practice was no longer viable. He sought other methods of obtaining an income and became the ready supplier of benzodiazepines and opiates for both the town's people and for other patients within 100 kilometres of his office.

His prescribing pattern was reported to the state Medical Council and he was requested to attend the council to discuss the matter. An appointment was made, the two interviewers were present, but Dr Abernethy failed to attend. He claimed illness. A second appointment was made for several weeks later, and Dr Abernethy failed to attend for the same reason. Investigations revealed that he was in fact seeing patients that day. He was strongly advised to attend at the next diarised appointment, which he did.

At that appointment it was obvious to the interviewers that Dr Abernethy was unable to think rationally, and they suggested it was time for him to retire. Dr Abernethy was highly indignant at this suggestion. He said that his wife had died, he had given his whole life to care for the local community, and that society owed him continuing employment because of his lifetime of service. The interviewers did not share his opinion.

They suggested that a senior general practitioner visit him to audit his practice. Dr Abernethy left in high dudgeon, only to return after 10 minutes to explain that he was unable to find his car in the small medical council car park. One of the secretaries assisted him to find his vehicle and he departed at high speed. In his haste he side-swiped the new car of one of the medical council staff. He did not stop when requested.

Doctor Abernethy sent a letter to the council two weeks later requesting that his name be removed from the register.

Legal Issues

The state Medical Council has two major responsibilities. The first is to protect the public from practitioners who are unable to cope with their professional responsibilities, and may cause patients harm. The second is to rehabilitate impaired practitioners, if they are likely to benefit from rehabilitation.

Discussion

It is a great difficulty for any individual, not just medical practitioners, to cope with their responsibilities at the end of their professional life, when they have devoted all their time to work and have not planned for retirement. As a general rule, those who actively plan the transition from full-time work cope better than those who are forced from full-time work without previous planning.

Clinical Principles

The problem that all practitioners face is acknowledging the need to retire when they know they are less able to cope. Fortunately most practitioners are aware of their limitations and act responsibly. If an impaired doctor lacks the insight to withdraw voluntarily from practice, the onus is on colleagues and others to advise the Medical Council.

MORAL IMPAIRMENT

History

Dr Edward Logan was a bulk billing general practitioner who invoiced Medicare for more than 30,000 services in one year. The quantum of billings led to investigation by the Professional Services Review (PSR), the body responsible for protection of the public purse.

When examined by a panel of his peers there were no medical records other than a date stamp referring to each time he had seen a patient. Dr Logan was unable to justify his billing and was required to reimburse the Commonwealth.

Legal Issues

Doctors are able to bill directly to the Commonwealth at a rate less than what they would receive if they adhered to the Australian Medical Association schedule of fees. Oversight exists via the PSR which holds outliers to account after they have been assessed by a panel of their peers. Errant practitioners may be required to reimburse the Commonwealth if they are found to be in breach of relevant regulations.

If practitioners appear twice before such a peer review panel (as a number have done) and are found to be noncompliant with the regulations, they are required to appear before a Medicare Participation Review Committee headed by a judge. This committee has the power to exclude the practitioner from access to Medicare payments.

Discussion

The bulk billing system is an honour system. Many practitioners believe that elimination of the need for detailed accounting leaves them more time to concentrate upon patient care. Others may seek to exploit the system fraudulently.

Clinical Principles

Appropriate billing and accurate accounting are necessary irrespective of Medicare. The vast majority of practitioners who bulk bill act responsibly and never come to the attention of a regulatory body.

Mechanisms are required to monitor billing and to identify and prosecute those who commit fraud.

SUBSTANCE ABUSE

History

Dr Stuart Chaucer, a respected practitioner in his community, had a surgical procedure, after which he was given multiple doses of pethidine over a four-day period. He became addicted and eventually came under the umbrella of the state Medical Council's impairment program.

Multiple conditions were placed on his practice (as per the council's protocol), including frequent urinalysis for narcotics, regular psychiatric, general practitioner and substance abuse practitioner attendances, and regular review by the council's assessors. After three years of supervision, with gradual reduction of conditions, he was allowed to resume independent practice, but was prohibited from prescribing or possessing narcotics.

Legal Issues

The state councils, in their role of protection of the public, have developed protocols over the years tailored to the needs of individual practitioners. Their power to enforce decisions relies on the provisions of the state Medical Practice Acts. Council protocols make it most unlikely for a medical practitioner with a known history of substance abuse to possess or prescribe narcotics.

Discussion

It is almost universal that practitioners who have been caught up in the maelstrom of substance abuse are relieved to be barred from possessing or prescribing these substances. Most express gratitude that the council imposed these restrictions on their ability to continue to practise.

Clinical Principles

The Medical Council restricts access by previous addicts to narcotics because of the risk of recidivism.

It is of interest to note that when Dr Chaucer was allowed to practise without the previously imposed sanctions, he wrote a letter to the interviewers thanking them for the dignified way in which they had managed his rehabilitation; stating that the council had saved his marriage, his sense of dignity and self-worth and his status in the eyes of his community.

PSYCHIATRIC IMPAIRMENT

HISTORY

Dr Bronte Dermott was a psychiatrist who became seriously mentally ill and attended the state Medical Council for an assessment. The interviewers were a very senior psychiatrist and a long-term member of the council. The conclusion reached at the meeting was that the doctor was impaired and a probable danger to his patients if he were to continue in practice. He was suspended from practice for one month with the obligation to urgently seek expert psychiatric care. The council would then review reports from the treating psychiatrist, and meet again with the impaired practitioner.

The state Medical Practice Act allowed for temporary suspension if it considered that continuing registration might cause harm to the practitioner's patients.

At the time of the initial interview, the senior psychiatrist was in the process of being appointed to the position of director of psychiatry in another state. Soon after the council interview, she took up her new appointment.

The impaired practitioner developed a personal grudge against the senior psychiatrist who had interviewed him. He pursued her interstate, discovered her whereabouts, and shot her dead.

He was soon arrested. In his wallet was a sketch plan of the residence of the other interviewer, with the doors, entrances and exits all clearly marked. The second interviewer was obviously to be the next victim.

LEGAL ISSUES

The practitioner was subject to the provisions of the state Supreme Court and now resides in the mental health unit of the prison system.

DISCUSSION

This doctor was self-managing his psychiatric condition, with no insight as to how this should be achieved, and no oversight from a colleague.

CLINICAL PRINCIPLES

Mental illness is present amongst medical practitioners, as well as in the general population. This case illustrates the need for medical practitioners to receive expert medical and mental health care for themselves, just as it is the case for the general population.

There is a legal requirement in Australia that all registered practitioners have their own treating general practitioner. If Dr Dermott had been managed by a competent general practitioner, he would likely have been referred sooner to a psychiatrist who may have been able to treat Dr Dermott effectively, and may have been able to ameliorate the risk of harm to Dr Dermott and others.

DECEPTION

HISTORY

Dr Aditya Banerjee, a recent medical graduate from Asia, travelled to Australia for postgraduate training. He found lodgings in the home of a family formerly from his home country. The host family lived close to his Australian training hospital.

Dr Banerjee went back to his country of origin for a vacation. On his return he approached Karima, the teenage daughter of his host family, when her parents were absent. He informed her that a number of infectious diseases were endemic in their country of birth, and that it would be wise for her to be immunised as a precautionary measure. Karima agreed to be immunised.

Dr Banerjee then injected her with a stupefying agent and took advantage of her on several occasions, topping up the medication as required. When he finished he dressed her modestly and left the house. Karima, on awakening, felt uncomfortable and complained to her mother who had by now returned home. Her general practitioner confirmed that she had been sexually abused. She had never previously had any intimate experience.

Dr Banerjee was interviewed by police and denied knowledge of any unlawful conduct. The police discovered a video recording of the whole sordid episode. The video was to be a trophy for him to use for his future enjoyment and to impress his friends.

Dr Banerjee was charged with drug administration without consent, acts of indecency and sexual intercourse without consent. He was suspended by the Medical Council, found guilty by the Supreme Court, and sentenced to a lengthy period of imprisonment. Following his release from prison he is to be deported to his country of origin with no opportunity to ever return to Australia or to be able to practise medicine in the future. The registration authority in his home country was informed of his conduct. Dr Banerjee will never be able to practise medicine there either.

INAPPROPRIATE EXAMINATION

HISTORY

Fiona Rail, a 32 year old hairdresser attended Dr Ned Black, her usual general practitioner, because of a problem with her three-year-old daughter. At the end of the consultation about her daughter, Fiona sought advice from Dr Black about skin lesions. Dr Black examined her lower limbs, commented on her attire and performed an inappropriate quick palpation of her clothed pelvic area.

Fiona was embarrassed by Dr Black's behaviour and commenced to leave the room when he made the comment that she caused him to be sexually aroused.

In a discussion between Fiona and her lawyer, from whom she sought advice, Fiona revealed that Dr Black had frequently pressured her to undergo an intimate examination that was not due at the time. She always refused these requests. The matter was examined by the Medical Council and Dr Black was deregistered.

VOYEURISM

History

Jennifer Rogers, aged 36 years, developed an inguinal hernia. Surgical correction was delayed because of a pregnancy. Eight weeks following delivery, and three weeks following hernia repair surgery, Dr Sam Spalding examined the hernia repair while Jennifer was lying down, but not while she was standing up. Following this, he examined her abdomen.

Dr Spalding then asked Jennifer to lie prone and lower her underpants, ostensibly to examine the epidural site, even though eight weeks had passed since delivery and there were no symptoms related to the epidural anaesthetic. He placed his hand on her bare buttocks during the examination and did not allow her any privacy while she was dressing, observing her all the while.

Jennifer felt violated by the doctor's behaviour and sought legal redress. He was interviewed by the Medical Council. Strict conditions were placed on his ability to practise.

Legal Issues

The final three brief examples raise several profound ethical and legal issues.

The case of Karima relates to conduct of the most grievous kind; conduct that must not be tolerated, and must be severely punished, as occurred in this case. The behaviour of this doctor breached one of the fundamental principles of medicine, to first do not harm.

The behaviour of Dr Black illustrates an ethical principle that has long been accepted across international boundaries and cultures. That is, the notion of affording the patient dignity.

The physical examination by Dr Spalding illustrates how careful the practitioner must be in his dealings with patients so as to not cause embarrassment or distress. Was he a voyeur or merely clinically careless? The investigation found that his behaviour was malevolent, and his practice was restricted accordingly.

None of the three doctors were sued in civil proceedings, although they could have been. Apart from Karima's case, the quantum of damages able to be recovered may have resulted in lawyers thinking litigation would be uncommercial. Many states have enacted legislation making it prohibitive to litigate small cases. The legal costs a defendant is obliged to pay a successful plaintiff are capped. A plaintiff may win but have her damages significantly eroded by her own legal costs including the cost of expert witnesses. In the circumstances, prosecution by something like the New South Wales Health

Care Complaints Commission (or even the police) may be the only available avenue to obtain justice.

Discussion

Ethical behaviour is that which ought to be done in a given situation, all things considered. A practitioner who adheres to this is unlikely to face litigation.

In all professions there are accepted standards of behaviour. These standards are well taught during the training period, and reinforced in the early stages of practice. The standards apply throughout practising life, and are fundamental to the practice of medicine. A doctor is in the privileged position of a close and intimate relationship with the patient, not only by virtue of knowledge of the patient's personal history, but also by virtue of the doctor's clinical examination.

At medical school, students are taught how to conduct examinations of all systems. Some examinations, such as respiratory and cardiac examinations, may require a female patient's bra to be removed. The proper examination of other systems may involve digital rectal or vaginal examinations. In a number of cases, we have found that these examinations are either omitted or, in the case of cardiac and respiratory examinations, carried out over clothing. Some practitioners either do not have the time or the inclination to be thorough. That is no reason to avoid performing what are uncomfortable or even embarrassing assessments for patients. But they must be done with proper regard to human dignity and with safeguards in place to ensure that a doctor's actions are not misinterpreted.

The origin of the phrase '*primum non nocere*' (first do no harm) is uncertain. Some attribute it to Galen, the 2nd century philosopher, whilst others dispute that origin. It was certainly well known in the 19th century. It exhorts the medical practitioner to refrain from causing harm to the patient whose medical condition he/she has the privilege of managing. Violating personal boundaries, especially those of vulnerable women who may have been abused in the past, can do considerable harm.

Another principle of medical practice is the notion of affording the patient dignity. This principle has been expressed in medical literature since antiquity:

> *'Whatever houses I may visit, I will come for the benefit of the sick, remaining free of all intentional injustice, of all mischief.' Oath of Hippocrates, c 400 BC;*
>
> *'Thou shall not commit adultery even in thought.' Oath of Initiation c 100 AD;*
>
> *'And you shall not lust after beautiful women.' Oath of Asaph c 600 AD; and*
>
> *'He should not look upon women with lust.' Advice to a physician c 900 AD.*

There are more references to dignity such as those from 1617 in China, Persia in 1770, Egypt in 1793, the American Medical Association in 1847, The Venezuelan Code of Medical Ethics 1918, The Declaration of Geneva

World Medical Association 1948 and The International Code of Medical Ethics 1949.

The doctor must be scrupulous in his dealings with patients so as to maintain ethical boundaries. At least in the case of Dr Spalding, if he had taken the simple precaution of asking a female employee to be present during the consultation, the problem may have been avoided.

Clinical Principles

There is no place for Hippocratic hypocrisy in the practice of medicine. There was no justification for the behaviours of any of these doctors. Patients are potentially vulnerable, and there is an imbalance of power between the doctor and the patient. Patient dignity must be respected at all times. And first do no harm.

References

All the quotations come from the Encyclopedia of Bioethics, McMillan and Free Press, 1978, p 1731 et seq.

POST-TRAUMATIC STRESS DISORDER

HISTORY

Gabrielle Dowling was born in 1985. At a young age, she was exposed to significant marital disharmony involving verbal and physical abuse. Ultimately, Gabrielle's father left the house and Gabrielle was brought up by her mother and grandmother. Her mother suffered from a number of medical conditions and at best provided intermittent support for her children. Gabrielle had two other siblings.

Between the ages of eight and twelve, Gabrielle was sexually abused by her grandmother's boyfriend. Later, as an adolescent, Gabrielle developed an eating disorder, anxiety and depression. Her pattern of eating was one of dietary restriction with episodes of purging, vomiting and obsessive exercising. On occasions, she felt disassociated and remote from events around her. Gabrielle used her eating disorder as a way to control her anxiety. She also started self-harming at an early age by cutting her arms and legs. She was diagnosed as having post-traumatic stress disorder (PTSD).

Despite her eating disorders, Gabrielle performed reasonably well at school and gained admission to a university to study journalism. However, she frequently suffered bouts of major depression with suicidal ideation, and attempted to take her life by overdoses on two occasions. She also developed drug and alcohol abuse. Inevitably, her psychiatric conditions interfered with her education. Gabrielle was not able to complete her degree.

She had lengthy admissions to both public and private psychiatric units. During one of her admissions to a private psychiatric unit, Gabrielle came under the care of Dr Ignatius Chung, who held himself out as an expert in the management of eating disorders. Dr Chung remained Gabrielle's treating psychiatrist for two years.

Dr Chung was a controlling and manipulative man. He insisted that Gabrielle follow his rules of practice. She had to cut off ties to family members; she had to provide him with her mobile phone number so that he could communicate with her at any time; and she had to keep the details of their therapy sessions confidential. He told her that if she broke any of the rules, he would cease to be her psychiatrist.

Gabrielle first saw Dr Chung in group sessions. The relationship then progressed to private sessions while an inpatient at the psychiatric unit. The sessions were often after hours with the door shut and locked. They were frequently impromptu. Sometimes, the consultations would last more than two hours. Dr Chung dimmed the light in the consulting room and moved close to Gabrielle. His physical proximity increased incrementally over the course of their therapeutic relationship. He began to put his legs on the outside of Gabrielle's legs so that they were in between his legs with her knees close to Dr Chung's genitals. He stroked her inner thigh and asked her intrusive questions about her sexual habits and her sex life. The sessions frequently involved touching and stroking other parts of her body.

Dr Chung sent personal text messages to Gabrielle and expected the same in reply. Dr Chung's unusual practices did not go unnoticed. Nursing staff at the psychiatric unit were aware of the manner in which Dr Chung conducted his sessions with Gabrielle, but did not do anything to intervene. His colleagues thought he was weird, and speculated among themselves about what he did, but left him alone.

Dr Chung's practices had the effect of reminding Gabrielle of her past abuse. This was comparable to being retraumatised. In addition, due to the profound loss of trust in the medical profession, Gabrielle felt isolated and without hope. She suffered from recurrent intrusive distressing memories of traumatic events, recurrent distressing dreams, dissociative reactions, and intense psychological distress at exposure to cues associated with past traumatic events. She developed a persistent low mood, with diminished interest to participate in activities, and a level of hypervigilance that left her continually looking for further negative life events.

Gabrielle's medical condition deteriorated while under Dr Chung's care. She attempted suicide by an overdose. Her weight dropped further. She was admitted to an intensive care unit and received parenteral nutrition.

Eventually, Dr Chung's practices were exposed and Gabrielle's treatment was transferred to another psychiatrist. She continues to suffer from a severe aggravation of PTSD and a major depressive disorder.

Legal Issues

Gabrielle commenced proceedings against Dr Chung and the company responsible for the private psychiatric unit in 2014, because of the post-traumatic stress she suffered as a result of Dr Chung's behaviour. Dr Chung did not contest the allegations of negligence made against him. The psychiatric unit argued that it could not reasonably have been aware of Dr Chung's practices as he was a private practitioner and it was not up to the psychiatric unit to tell a private consultant how to conduct his therapy sessions.

Despite these arguments, the matter settled at mediation.

Discussion

This case highlights the importance of setting boundaries between a medical practitioner and patient. Boundary violations can take many forms. They can entail a degree of familiarity more appropriate between friends or family members, in which cases objectivity may be lost and important diagnoses missed. At the other end of the scale, there may be sexual intercourse or assault. Dr Chung engaged in gross boundary violations to the detriment of Gabrielle's health.

In order to ameliorate the risk of boundary violations, it is generally accepted that a practitioner needs to be aware that boundary violations can occur, and to appreciate that some patients are at greater risk than others. In psychiatric practice, the risk is high, as exemplified by Gabrielle's case. To protect against this risk, there is often a need for clinical supervision of therapy sessions and a clear understanding of the roles of the practitioner in the treatment of the patient.

Psychotherapy supervision is required in order to protect not only the patient, but also the therapist from becoming too enmeshed with the patient's life. It provides assistance in dealing with patients who have complex or especially challenging problems, addressing ethical concerns and boundary issues.

A boundary represents the limit of appropriate behaviour by a psychiatrist or other professional in the clinical setting. There is a need for no physical contact, circumscribed lengths of appointment, confidentiality and avoidance of social or personal relationships. There should be no self-disclosure by the clinician and there should be a specific location where the clinical contact should take place. Not all therapeutic relationships need to have this level of supervision. Simple steps such as having a nurse present during an examination or a third person in a consultation may be all that is necessary.

Although Dr Chung did not engage in sexual intercourse with Gabrielle, he nonetheless violated the doctor–patient boundary in a physical and sexually suggestive manner. There is a well-established connection between eating disorders and sexual abuse. Dr Chung's treatment unsurprisingly aggravated all of Gabrielle's underlying psychopathologies.

The case also highlights the importance of the role of nursing staff in the management of hospitalised patients. Despite the nurses' view that they should not interfere in the management of Gabrielle's condition by Dr Chung, that was precisely the response required by nursing staff in the circumstances. Nursing staff spend more time with inpatients than doctors. Their insights into the health and wellbeing of patients should not be underestimated. Doctors should listen to the opinions of nursing staff about the management of their patients. In Gabrielle's case, more forthright involvement by nursing staff likely would have stopped Dr Chung's damaging practices sooner.

Clinical Principles

Eating disorders are complex conditions that require an appreciation of the association with past sexual abuse and the danger of boundary violations to both practitioner and patient. There are guidelines for the avoidance of boundary violations of which all practitioners should be cognisant, especially psychiatrists.

DELIRIUM

HISTORY

Ruby Chen was born in 1973. On 20 April 2005, at the age of 31, Ruby gave birth to a daughter by caesarean section. At the time of the birth, Ruby was a successful veterinary surgeon. She had abused benzodiazepines and alcohol in the past. She frequently travelled to Papua New Guinea (PNG) in the course of her work.

The day after delivery, Ruby developed an acute delirium. At 10:50 h, she was noted to appear tired and to have slow, slurred speech. Later that morning Ruby left her baby unattended, and was again observed to have slurred speech. At 16:00 h, Ruby was agitated and defensive when questioned about her condition. Her speech was still slurred and nursing staff thought she was affected by drugs. She denied taking any illicit substances or any prescription medication other than that which the hospital had administered.

One hour later, Ruby was noted to be confused, incoherent and again to have slurred speech. Staff again thought she had taken drugs. The basis of their thinking was Ruby's past history of benzodiazepine and alcohol abuse. Nobody attached significance to her work history of frequent trips to PNG.

Nursing staff at the hospital thought she had smuggled diazepam and temazepam into the hospital. Ruby again denied this suggestion. That evening, Ruby was noted to be uncooperative and unsteady on her feet, repeatedly trying to get out of bed. Her Glasgow Coma Scale score (GCS) decreased to 13/15 and her oxygen saturation was 94% (reference >95%). She was hypotensive with a blood pressure of 95/50 mmHg.

At 19:30 h on 20 April 2005, Ruby was reviewed by the medical registrar, who considered the likely diagnosis was an overdose of benzodiazepines, despite Ruby's protestations that she had not taken any. He ordered transfer to the high dependency unit for the administration of midazolam for sedation. Neither blood nor urinary drug screening was performed. Ruby was then reviewed by the psychiatry registrar, who also considered she had a delirium secondary to benzodiazepine abuse.

The next morning, Ruby was reviewed by the consultant psychiatrist. He also thought she was suffering from an acute delirium secondary to benzodiazepines, but considered it necessary to exclude intracranial pathology. He ordered a CT scan of Ruby's brain without contrast. The scan was reported as showing no abnormality, although in retrospect it in fact demonstrated a left cerebellar hemispheric abnormality.

By 27 April 2005, the acute delirium had resolved and Ruby was discharged from hospital with her new baby.

One month afterwards, Ruby presented to the emergency department at the same hospital for advice and treatment in relation to headaches, lethargy and general malaise since her discharge. Medical staff in the emergency department elicited a history of delirium shortly after caesarean section delivery together with a past history of benzodiazepine and alcohol abuse. Ruby was diagnosed as suffering from an anxiety neurosis and discharged home to be further managed by her general practitioner.

Less than one month later in June 2005, Ruby was admitted as an involuntary patient to a psychiatric unit at a nearby hospital because of increasingly disorganised behaviour and threats of self-harm. She was diagnosed with benzodiazepine dependence, postpartum depression and a borderline personality disorder.

On 23 June 2005, a further CT scan of Ruby's brain was ordered. The appearances were suggestive of meningitis. Ruby was transferred to a tertiary hospital, where she underwent a lumbar puncture. Cerebrospinal fluid (CSF) from the lumbar puncture was positive for cryptococcal antigen. Culture of the CSF grew cryptococci. As a result, Ruby was diagnosed with cryptococcal meningoencephalitis. She was commenced on treatment with fluconazole and then voriconazole.

Ruby made a gradual recovery, but was left with neuropsychological deficits, including mild to moderate deficits in executive function and memory. She also developed hydrocephalus and required the insertion of an external ventricular drain on 13 July 2005. She claimed to have developed an adjustment disorder with depressed mood as a result of the meningitis.

Legal Issues

In 2009, Ruby commenced proceedings against the local area health service responsible for the hospital at which she delivered her baby and to which she subsequently presented one month after discharge. She sued the health service in negligence for failing adequately to exclude intracranial pathology before diagnosing her with benzodiazepine abuse, an anxiety neurosis and depression.

She alleged that, in light of her work history, staff should have thought of unusual infections as the cause of her delirium. Finally, she alleged that a CT scan of the brain without contrast was an inadequate means of excluding cerebral pathology such as an infection.

Ruby alleged that, if the diagnosis had been made earlier, and proper treatment instituted, she would have made a complete or near complete recovery and would have avoided her ongoing cognitive and neuropsychiatric sequelae.

Ruby relied on the expert evidence of two psychiatrists, a neurologist and two infectious diseases physicians. The defendant had a similar array of expert evidence refuting Ruby's claim. Although Ruby obtained the opinion of a neuroradiologist in relation to the interpretation of the CT scan without contrast, it was accepted that an ordinary skilled radiologist would not necessarily have been able to identify the cerebellar abnormalities on the CT scan of 22 April 2005.

The matter went to two mediations and eventually settled prior to a hearing.

Discussion

The critical question in this case was whether it was reasonable to attribute Ruby's acute delirium to a psychiatric cause, including drug withdrawal or intoxication, without first excluding a neurological or other organic cause. This question also arose in relation to the subsequent presentation to the emergency department at the hospital about one month after discharge. The subsidiary question was whether a CT scan of the brain without contrast was an appropriate means of excluding alternative diagnoses.

The consultant psychiatrist at the hospital clearly thought it necessary to exclude an organic cause for the acute delirium despite nursing staff being quick to ascribe Ruby's delirium to benzodiazepines. This is why he ordered a CT scan. There was no question that, as a screening test for intracerebral pathology, a CT scan of the brain without contrast was a reasonable first step, but further steps were required. The infectious diseases physicians and neurologists relied on by Ruby said that, in circumstances where an infective cause needed to be excluded, especially given her travel to PNG, it was unreasonable to rely only on a CT scan without contrast.

The defendant's neurology and infectious diseases experts argued that a CT scan without contrast was all that was required and that it was appropriate to make a provisional or working diagnosis of benzodiazepine intoxication or withdrawal. Cryptococcosis was so rare that it could be ignored as a sensible differential diagnosis.

Whether it was reasonable at that time or at the subsequent presentation to make a psychiatric diagnosis without first excluding an organic cause depends upon what differential diagnoses a reasonable neurologist ought to have made both in the acute phase after caesarean section delivery, and one month later in the emergency department. The experts on both sides agreed that the delirium could have been due to intracerebral pathology. It is known that a CT scan without contrast will not pick up all pathology. Given that infection was one of a number of reasonable differential diagnoses, an ordinary skilled neurologist should not have considered that all possibilities had been excluded simply by ordering a CT scan without contrast.

The case highlights the maxim that a practitioner should not make a psychiatric diagnosis until an organic cause has been reasonably excluded. Put shortly, an organic cause was considered, but not reasonably excluded.

It appears that the diagnosis of benzodiazepine intoxication or withdrawal became entrenched soon after triage. By the time Ruby presented one month after her initial discharge, staff in the emergency department were wedded to a psychiatric diagnosis and did not take the investigation of a possible organic cause any further. An opportunity to diagnose the cryptococcosis earlier was again missed.

The significant work history of travel to PNG should have been a red flag to potentially unusual causes of delirium. If cerebrospinal fluid had been taken in April 2005, it more likely than not would have detected cryptococcal antigen. The abnormality on the CT scan was made in retrospect. Given that it was likely to have been representative of meningitis, an earlier MRI scan would probably have detected the meningitis and led to screening for a range of possibilities, including cryptococcosis, given that this was tested for when the condition was ultimately diagnosed, and Ruby was a veterinary surgeon who frequently travelled to PNG.

This case highlights the importance of history-taking in making a diagnosis. If staff had listened to Ruby's denial of taking drugs, attached significance to her work history and appreciated that an acute delirium pointed to an organic cause, the diagnosis was much more likely to have been made sooner.

Clinical Principles

Cryptococcal meningitis is an uncommon disease. There are many causes of meningitis, but the symptoms of most cases of meningitis are similar and, once suspected, should be investigated by way of lumbar puncture and appropriate neuroimaging.

An emergency department doctor or a neurologist being asked to review a patient in the obstetric ward may not have known all of the rare causes of meningitis, such as cryptococcosis. However, the pattern of symptoms and signs were indicative of possible meningitis, and a lumbar puncture ought to have been performed.

FAMILY DYNAMICS

History

Rohan Kirkup was a 79-year-old man who lived alone following the admission of his wife to a nursing home one year previously. He had two daughters – Chris, who was said to have had a long-standing history of substance abuse, and Anne. Anne lived close-by and Chris several hours away. Chris visited from time to time. Rohan was friendly with his next-door neighbour, a man of age similar to him. Significant pressure was placed upon him by both of his daughters to move to a retirement complex close to his wife's accommodation. He was unwilling to do this at that time, as he believed that he was able to cope independently, and he was suspicious of their motivation. He did not intend to take that step for a number of years.

Rohan's health status had two adverse features, these being a history of epilepsy since 1974 for which he had been treated with phenytoin, and atrial fibrillation (AF) for which he was anticoagulated with warfarin. His epilepsy had been well controlled until six months prior to these events when he was changed from phenytoin to topiramate, following which he developed severe psychiatric symptoms. These symptoms resolved when he was changed back to phenytoin.

On 23 September Anne took her father to his general practitioner, Dr Simon Geraty, who felt that Rohan was in his usual state of health and that he did not require any change of medication. There was no record of any psychiatric examination. Anne visited her father the next day. Rohan had not allowed her into his house, saying that he believed that his wife's jewellery had been stolen and he would not let anyone into the house.

Anne was concerned about her father and attended Dr Geraty. Dr Geraty, who had not previously considered Rohan to be psychiatrically ill, completed a form for involuntary admission to an acute psychiatric facility. The form stated that Dr Geraty assessed Rohan to be "paranoid and cognitively impaired" based on his supposed observation of "abnormalities of behaviour and conduct observed by myself". The difficulty in which Dr Geraty found himself related to the fact that he had not seen Rohan on the day he completed the admission form.

Rohan, unwilling to go to hospital, was collected by the police, who conveyed him to the acute psychiatric facility. The admitting doctor at the hospital merely copied the notes from the general practitioner's referral. She did not conduct any independent assessment.

Following his admission to the hospital Anne went on her planned two-week holiday to another state.

Rohan displayed what appeared to be paranoid ideation at the hospital and this was recorded on multiple occasions. The psychiatric registrar wrote, "Was outwardly settled but pressured and tangential ?paranoid and rambling about daughters trying to take money. Difficult to assess if this is a valid fear or a paranoid idea." His ideation in fact was related to his well-founded belief that his daughters were attempting to induce him to sell his house for their financial gain and that one of them had stolen his wife's jewellery.

The nurse's record of the same day indicated that Rohan was angry with what they were doing in "putting me in here and trying to take my money". There was a further notation by the psychiatric registrar of "nil evidence of paranoid beliefs in any other area".

After a week in hospital Rohan was assessed by a consultant psychiatrist. The mini-mental score was 26 out of 30 and Addenbrooke's cognitive examination score was 83%, both of which were appropriate values for a 79-year-old. The psychiatrist observed that Rohan had tangential thinking with some fixed ideas of a paranoid nature, but not sufficient to be labelled as mentally ill. Rohan was discharged home.

His trusted next-door neighbour, at a later date, discovered Rohan's wife's jewellery in the window of the local pawnbrokers.

Legal Issues

Rohan took legal action against the general practitioner and the hospital. He sued in negligence and for false imprisonment.

Opinions were obtained from general practitioner and psychiatric experts. There was no support for Dr Geraty's baseless scheduling of Rohan as an involuntary patient. He should have assessed him properly and taken into account Rohan's views about his daughters' conduct. There was likewise no support for the hospital's conduct by the employed psychiatric registrar. She should have performed an independent examination rather than repeating Dr Geraty's flawed assessment. The damages claimed were not great, but that did not mean that the wrongfulness of the conduct could be ignored.

The case settled at mediation. Rohan will be able to direct the distribution of his estate in due course according to his wishes.

Discussion

This was a classic example of elder abuse and raises many issues.

Dr Geraty did not believe Rohan to be psychiatrically impaired one day, yet accepted the word of Anne the next day and recorded that Rohan was impaired. It was wrong to request involuntary admission to a psychiatric facility without further objective assessment.

The admitting junior doctor at the hospital did not record any independent assessment. This was inexcusable.

Rohan was not assessed by a consultant psychiatrist until the seventh day following his admission, contrary to pertinent legislation. Psychiatric review is mandated within five days after involuntary admission.

Rohan's assertion that his daughters were trying to disadvantage him was not given credence by the various medical professionals, and he was essentially incarcerated unjustly without adequate assessment and against his will.

This case illustrates the importance of thorough assessment of a patient, particularly an elderly patient who may be suffering from early dementia, prior to depriving him of his liberty. Elderly patients may take longer to assess. This is not an excuse to cut corners or carry out superficial assessments.

The case also illustrates how vulnerable patients, particularly elderly patients, may be abused by scheming family members who are intent on disadvantaging them.

Regrettably, children do not always act in the best interest of their parents. It was fortunate that Rohan had an astute neighbour who was able to affirm that Rohan's version of the story was correct.

Clinical Principles

Psychiatric assessment requires a structured approach including careful personal examination of the patient. It requires patience. It is never enough to take the word of potentially biased third parties. The assessment needs to take into account the age and social circumstances of a patient.

The law requires that an individual cannot be detained involuntarily for more than five days in a psychiatric facility without consultant psychiatric assessment.

CEREBRAL PALSY

HISTORY

Hayley was born on 4 July 2006. She was the first child of Grace and Anthony Campbell. Grace became pregnant with Hayley in the second half of 2005. The estimated date of birth by dates and ultrasound was 22 June 2006. Once the pregnancy was diagnosed, Grace's general practitioner referred her to the antenatal clinic at the nearby tertiary referral hospital for management of the pregnancy and subsequent labour and delivery.

Grace attended the antenatal clinic on 11 occasions. She and her baby remained in good condition throughout the pregnancy. All routine antenatal screening investigations were normal.

At 18:45 h on 3 July 2006, Grace was admitted to the labour ward at the hospital at gestation 41 weeks and 5 days, for induction of labour.

Labour was induced by the vaginal application of dinoprostone gel 10 mg, artificial rupture of membranes (ARM) the following day and an oxytocin infusion. At the time of the ARM, the cervix was dilated 1 cm and the presenting part (cephalic) was 3 cm above the ischial spines.

Labour commenced at about 12:05 h on 4 July 2006. In terms of cervical dilation and station of the presenting part, Grace's labour progressed as follows:

TIME (hr)	CERVICAL DILATION (cm)	STATION (cm) ABOVE/BELOW ISCHIAL SPINES
14:15	2	–2 to –3
16:15	2–3	–1 to –2
17:10	6	–1 to –2
20:30	10	0

Oxytocin was infused during the following periods at the following rates:

PERIOD (hr)	CONCENTRATION (U/L)	RATE (drops/min)
10:00–11:00	10	15
11:00–12:00	10	30
12:00–13:00	10	90
13:00–14:00	10	150
14:00–16:00	10	180
16:00–17:45	10	210

Continued

PERIOD (hr)	CONCENTRATION (U/L)	RATE (drops/min)
17:45–18:15	20	105
18:15–19:05	Infusion suspended	Nil
19:05–22:00	20	45
22:00–22:25	Infusion suspended	Nil
22:25–23:22	20	45

Fetal wellbeing and contractions were monitored by extended periods of cardiotocography (CTG) or with a fetal scalp electrode (FSE). From 16:50 h on 4 July 2006, the CTG demonstrated uterine tachysystole (more than 5 contractions every 10 minutes), and fetal heart rate (FHR) abnormalities of decreased beat-to-beat variability with variable decelerations. These abnormalities were present until 18:15 h on 4 July 2006. Thereafter, the following abnormalities were observable on the CTG:

PERIOD (hr)	ABNORMALITY
18:30–19:00	Decreased beat-to-beat variability
18:15–19:05	Normal beat-to-beat variability (oxytocin suspended)
19:05–21:00	Decreased beat-to-beat variability
21:00–22:00	Uterine hyperstimulation, decreased beat-to-beat variability, variable decelerations, increasing baseline FHR
22:00–22:25	FHR abnormalities persisted (oxytocin suspended)
22:25–22:50	Uterine hyperstimulation, decreased beat-to-beat variability, variable decelerations, fetal tachycardia
22:50–23:20	Uterine hyperstimulation, decreased beat-to-beat variability, variable and late decelerations, fetal tachycardia

Grace also developed pyrexia late in labour. At about 23:19 h, the midwives made a diagnosis of shoulder dystocia. Delivery was first attempted by using the McRoberts manoeuvre, and when this failed, the reverse Wood screw manoeuvre.

Hayley was delivered vaginally at 23:22 h on 4 July 2006. At delivery, she required immediate resuscitation because of the absence of a heart beat and respirations. She weighed 3,822 g and was acidotic (first cord pH 6.9, base excess minus 13.1 mEq/L). Her APGAR scores were 2 and 2 at one and five minutes of age.

Within 24 hours of her birth, Hayley was diagnosed with Sarnat stage 2 hypoxic ischaemic encephalopathy (HIE). She went on to develop a spastic quadriplegic cerebral palsy with dystonic features.

MRI scans of Hayley's brain demonstrated damage principally to the deep grey matter and basal ganglia, and some cortical signal changes. The pattern of injury was consistent with a severe, short period of hypoxia and ischaemia. Hayley suffered a cardiac arrest in utero, which logically must have been preceded by bradycardia. Her circulatory collapse was the consequence of evolving acidaemia as her reserves or defence mechanisms were depleted and ultimately failed.

Legal Issues

In 2009, Hayley commenced legal proceedings against the local area health service responsible for the negligence of the midwives and medical practitioners who managed the labour and delivery. Due to her age and disabilities, Hayley brought the proceedings by a tutor, her mother. The tutor was charged with the responsibility for making decisions during the litigation in Hayley's best interests. Such decisions included whether to proceed to a hearing or to settle out of court.

Liability was contested in relation to both breach of duty and causation of damage. The plaintiff relied on the expert evidence of a midwife and three obstetricians. The defendant qualified a single expert, an obstetrician, who argued that the labour was properly managed. He considered any FHR abnormalities on the CTG were identified and acted upon promptly. The oxytocin infusion was titrated in accordance with accepted practice, and the uterine tachysystole was correctly remedied by slowing the rate of the oxytocin infusion.

The case was settled at mediation in accordance with the tutor's instructions. The settlement was subsequently approved by the Supreme Court as being reasonable and in Hayley's best interests.

Discussion

The central allegation was that the hospital's midwives and junior obstetric staff essentially failed to recognise the evolving seriousness of Hayley's condition. This, in turn, raised questions about the quality of training in the application, interpretation and use of FHR monitoring during labour. In this case, it was alleged that staff misinterpreted the CTG trace, and persisted with the oxytocin infusion in the presence of a nonreassuring FHR pattern on the CTG. Early vaginal delivery was likely possible given the rates of descent of the presenting part, and cervical dilation.

The staff should have recognised that the FHR trace was abnormal, abandoned oxytocin, arranged for Grace and Hayley to be reviewed by a senior obstetrics registrar or obstetrician, and expedited delivery. Instead, staff managed the labour conservatively, particularly during the second stage (from 20:30 h) when there was no basis for inaction in light of the persistent and suspicious FHR abnormalities.

In other obstetrics cases, the FHR abnormalities are recognised and thought sufficiently important to immediately influence clinical decisions.

Why did those caring for Grace and Hayley attach no significance to the FHR abnormalities they observed?

The collective view of the plaintiff's experts was that a decision to deliver should have been made at 22:15 h. Delivery at this time was achievable vaginally because the second stage of labour had commenced at 20:30 h. If this had occurred then Hayley would have been delivered 22:30–22:40 h at the latest.

The defendant relied on one obstetric witness. His opinion was completely at odds with the opinions of the three other obstetric experts. Surprisingly, he was not supplied with the CTG up to 19:00 h on 4 July 2006 and so was unaware of the nonreassuring or ominous FHR patterns before the oxytocin was first turned off. While he acknowledged that there were decelerations and decreased variability, he considered it reasonable to have monitored the trace rather than to have interfered and expedited delivery. He said it was reasonable to ascribe the fetal tachycardia to Grace's pyrexia. He accepted that this opinion was in hindsight and that it was unsafe to attribute it to maternal pyrexia at the time.

The plaintiff relied on paediatric neurology, neonatology and paediatric neuroradiological opinion to support causation. The hospital also relied on a neonatology opinion and a neuroradiologist. There was little difference in the interpretation of the imaging. The dispute centred on whether Hayley would have avoided all or a significant part of her permanent brain damage with delivery 40 to 50 minutes prior to her actual delivery.

It was unlikely that Hayley would have avoided all her brain damage, but she would have been significantly better off with earlier delivery. There was a serious dispute about the amount she should recover in damages. As is usual in cerebral palsy cases, there was an argument about life expectancy, since life expectancy has a significant impact on the damages available to a plaintiff.

Clinical Principles

The case highlights a common failing in obstetrics cases at public hospitals – lack of involvement of more senior staff. The plaintiff relied on the opinions of two professors of obstetrics, a general obstetrician and a registered midwife. Their evidence was that the FHR abnormalities and uterine tachysystole were clearly related to the oxytocin, as these abnormalities disappeared promptly when the oxytocin was ceased at 18:15 h, but returned when it was restarted at 19:05 h. In addition, the FHR abnormalities persisted when the oxytocin was turned off for the second time at 22:00 h (i.e. fetal distress persisted despite suspension of oxytocin on this occasion).

There was no conceivable basis for restarting the oxytocin at 22:25 h in light of the obvious connection between its use and signs of fetal compromise. All of these red flags would have been identified and acted upon by a senior obstetrics registrar or obstetrician if present or if called at 22:00 h when the FHR abnormalities persisted despite switching off the oxytocin infusion.

The registered midwife expert was able to identify the abnormalities on the CTG, and was of the opinion that the hospital's midwifery staff should also have been able to detect the problems and call for obstetrics help. The expert obstetricians thought that a decision to deliver should have been made by 22:45 h at the latest.

The system may encourage these types of outcomes by placing too much reliance on junior staff, who do not have experience with impending catastrophes. It cannot be good obstetric practice to wait until there is a blindingly obvious abnormality before calling in the senior specialists. Junior members of the team must not only be educated on technical matters relevant to the discipline in which they are currently working, but also encouraged to develop skills to recognise their limitations and be forthright in asking for the help of senior colleagues.

TOXOPLASMOSIS

In this chapter, we describe two cases of toxoplasmosis to highlight the importance of accurate diagnosis and early treatment.

UNWELL AT ROUTINE PREGNANCY CHECK

HISTORY

When Camilla Torrington was seven weeks pregnant she presented to her general practitioner, Dr Mariam Bonnici, for her first prenatal consultation. Camilla told Dr Bonnici that she had swollen glands in the neck as well as other mild symptoms. Dr Bonnici ordered tests for toxoplasmosis that demonstrated that Camilla had suffered from this disease at some time in her life, maybe in the past, maybe currently. The pathologist requested that the test be repeated in two weeks to determine whether or not the titre was rising, thus indicating a recent infection. This repeat test was not performed and the potential significance of the clinical symptoms was lost. Camilla was seen by a different doctor later in her pregnancy, and was not reviewed by Dr Bonnici.

All went well until delivery and for several subsequent weeks. Baby Florence developed an array of disabilities. Investigations revealed *Toxoplasma gondii* DNA within Florence's cerebrospinal fluid. Florence now has hydrocephalus, seizures, global development delay, diabetes insipidus, hypothyroidism and visual impairment due to chorioretinitis.

LEGAL ISSUES

Camilla sought compensation from Dr Torrington on behalf of her daughter for the injuries caused by the failure to diagnose and treat toxoplasmosis in early pregnancy.

There was no dispute about the cause of Florence's disabilities or that she would probably have avoided them if toxoplasmosis had been diagnosed and treated in early pregnancy. The issue addressed by expert general practitioners was whether Dr Torrington's conduct constituted appropriate practice for review of test results.

The general practitioner for the plaintiff argued that the positive result in the context of the enlarged lymph nodes should have resulted in further testing with recall of Camilla if needed. The general practitioner engaged by the defendant argued that a significant proportion of the general population will test positively for toxoplasma. Camilla's symptoms and signs were non-specific and mild. He thought no further action was required. There was no evidence of other possible features of toxoplasmosis including jaundice, rash or hepatosplenomegaly.

The case is ongoing.

Discussion

This problem arose because a pathology test was not followed up. Dr Bonnici ordered the test and did not record on the medical record that Camilla had swollen lymph nodes. A second doctor from the same practice saw Camilla at the subsequent consultation and it seems that she also did not review the pathology results and comments. By the time the second doctor saw Camilla, it was too late to avoid the outcome. For this reason, she was not joined as a defendant. This does not mean her practice should be condoned.

There were several confounding factors, one of which was that there were two practitioner partners involved in the management of Camilla. Another was that Camilla lived in an Australian State where toxoplasmosis testing was unavailable. Her blood sample was sent to a national reference laboratory. The result, when it was finally received, was either lost, not understood or was not even viewed by the two practitioners. Whatever did occur, the result was not passed on to Camilla and baby Florence paid a great price.

Doctors must ensure that procedures are established and followed to ensure that test results are not only viewed but also signed off by a doctor. Ideally this should be done by the doctor who ordered the test. If an abnormal test is reviewed by a different doctor, then the requesting doctor should be advised of the result.

Contemporary general practitioner software programs do not allow results to be stored until they have been viewed. Options thereafter usually include no action, or urgent recall.

Clinical Principles

Toxoplasma antibodies are commonly found in the general population without there being any clinical symptoms or signs. Exposure to toxoplasma is often associated with contact with cats, months or years before antibodies are detected.

Women infected before conception ordinarily do not transmit it to the fetus. The condition is dangerous when it occurs in early pregnancy because there is a ~15% transmission rate to the fetus. The presence of toxoplasmosis can be best assessed by polymerase chain reaction analysis of amniotic fluid for the B1 gene of *Toxoplasma gondii*. Specific treatment is indicated for acute toxoplasmosis of newborns, pregnant women and immunocompromised patients.

In France, Austria and some USA states pregnant women and/or newborns are routinely screened for toxoplasmosis. This is not the case in Australia.

BABY WITH LARGE LIVER

HISTORY

Baby Damian was found to have a congenital cardiac abnormality at birth, for which he received urgent surgery. After 14 days an enlarged liver was detected. There were no other features to suggest cardiac failure, and it was correctly assumed that the hepatomegaly was not related to the congenital heart disease. Over the following year hepatomegaly 3–8 cm was found on several occasions by different general practitioners at the local medical centre. Both of Damian's parents were intellectually impaired and lived in a state of domestic chaos. Damian failed to thrive and developed a number of abnormalities over the following months and years.

Damian was finally assessed by a paediatrician who found that he had toxoplasmosis. Damian, now profoundly disabled, is still in the care of his dysfunctional family.

LEGAL ISSUES

Once the paediatrician carefully explained the diagnosis and that the infection was probably present from birth, Damian's family sought compensation on his behalf for the consequences of delayed diagnosis and treatment of toxoplasmosis. Individuals such as Damian's parents may not seek compensation because they do not know where to start, or who can help them.

The hepatomegaly was never investigated despite a connection with the congenital cardiac abnormality having been ruled out very early. The general practitioner expert qualified by the family expressed the firm view that a reasonable general practitioner should have referred Damian to a paediatrician for assessment in the first year of his life. As Damian was reviewed by multiple practitioners, there was a long list of defendants.

The case is ongoing.

DISCUSSION

Although there was no evidence of cardiac failure following neonatal cardiac surgery, no investigation was initially performed to explain hepatomegaly. Toxoplasmosis was only diagnosed years later by which time Damian had permanent disabilities. The reason for the delay was unclear. The general practitioners may well have assumed that the cause or significance of the hepatomegaly had been excluded by the specialist team responsible for the cardiac surgery. One or more of the general practitioners may have thought a colleague had investigated the issue. It is never safe to make such assumptions. Contemporary record keeping should make it clear when a condition has or has not been investigated.

Damian's parents were unlikely to have been forthright advocates of their son's health. It is an unfortunate fact that first impressions may adversely influence management decisions. Doctors must be careful not to reduce their vigilance because an individual presents intellectually impaired, or unclean, or otherwise unusual. All patients should be afforded the best treatment available. Patients such as Damian have to rely on others and the expertise of the medical practitioner to ensure best care.

Clinical Principles

Toxoplasmosis can be treated, both in early pregnancy when the clinical features of an acute illness with swollen cervical glands lead to investigation, and in the newborn. Treatment is most often with pyrimethamine plus sulfadiazine or clindamycin. Corticosteroids are administered concurrently for retinochoroiditis.

POSTNATAL DEPRESSION

HISTORY

On 19 April 2012, at the age of 33, solicitor Amanda Gordon gave birth to her first child. She and her partner Phillip were excited about the pregnancy and birth after years of anguish with failed attempts at in vitro fertilisation. At the time she became pregnant, Amanda had no significant surgical, medical or family history. She had experienced an episode of minor anxiety and depression associated with her work. These symptoms settled with a short course of antidepressant medication.

The pregnancy was managed on a shared-care basis between her general practitioner and the antenatal clinic at a Sydney public hospital. There were no problems during the pregnancy. There were no problems with labour and delivery. Amanda and her newborn son, Angus, were discharged three days after delivery on 22 April 2012.

Five days later, Amanda presented to the emergency department at the hospital where she had delivered Angus, complaining of anxiety, suicidal thoughts, insomnia and a low mood. She was assessed by a mental health nurse practitioner and by a perinatal mental health nurse. Both obtained a history of high levels of anxiety, panic and hyperventilation, insomnia with racing thoughts, suicidal ideation, anorexia and a feeling of doom in the evening. Amanda's waves of anxiety were more severe than anything she had experienced before. She felt that she needed to be admitted to hospital. Despite these symptoms and her desire to be admitted to hospital, after review by the mental health nurse practitioner, Amanda was discharged from the emergency department and advised to re-present if her anxiety worsened or she had further thoughts of self-harm.

The next day, on 28 April 2012, the mental health nurse practitioner telephoned Amanda, who reported having had four hours sleep and feeling a bit better. He arranged for Amanda to be reviewed in the hospital by the psychiatric registrar two days later.

As events turned out, Amanda was unable to wait for the appointment on 30 April 2012. She presented by ambulance on 29 April 2012 after taking an overdose of 23 tablets of oxazepam 15 mg at 03:00 h that morning.

At presentation, a psychiatric registrar reviewed Amanda. He obtained a history of suicidal ideation, very poor sleep, no appetite, weight loss, a bleak mood, feelings of being a burden to her family and that they would be better off without her, intermittent periods of intense suicidal ideation, including the specific thought of driving into the wilderness and not returning.

The doctor also obtained a history of her previous episode of anxiety and depression.

On mental state examination, Amanda had psychomotor retardation, intermittent teariness, long reply latency and a restricted and dysphoric affect. He diagnosed Amanda as suffering from a major postnatal depressive disorder and assessed her as being at an increased risk of self-harm. She agreed to be admitted to the hospital's psychiatric unit as a voluntary patient, and was placed on level II observations (to be sighted by staff every 10 minutes).

After admission, Amanda was assessed by a consultant psychiatrist, who acknowledged the history taken by the registrar and advised the commencement of temazepam 10–20 mg at night for sedation and a tricyclic antidepressant, dothiepin, at a starting dose of 50 mg to be titrated up to 100 mg over the following week.

On 5 May 2012, Amanda was prescribed promethazine 10 mg for night sedation, which was increased two days later to 25 mg. She was also prescribed, from 1 May 2012, diazepam, 2–5 mg three times daily as necessary for anxiety.

During the course of her admission, Amanda's observation level was downgraded and she had increasing periods of escorted and then unescorted day leave. By 12 May 2012, she was authorised to have extended unescorted day leave. These changes reflected the psychiatric team's impression that Amanda's condition was improving. In fact, she continued to have poor, broken sleep, anxiety about returning home because it reminded her of the meltdown she experienced at the time of admission, and anxiety about being able to sleep.

When Amanda was allowed extended leave on 13 May 2012, nursing staff recorded that she was anxious about being given leave. Later that night at 21:30 h, after she returned from leave, nursing staff recorded that she had dark thoughts while on leave and that she had suicidal thoughts. She was noted to have a low mood with a restricted affect. Neither the psychiatrist nor psychiatric registrar were apprised of these developments.

At 08:00 h on 14 May 2012, Amanda was assessed by a psychiatric nurse, Mr Jacob Smith, as being suitable for unescorted day leave. At the time, Mr Smith was unaware of the history recorded in the notes at 21:30 h on 13 May 2012 or of Amanda's dark mood and suicidal intent. The history was omitted from the nursing handover that morning.

At some time on the morning of being granted unescorted leave, Amanda drove her car to the Blue Mountains National Park and threw herself over a cliff to her death.

Legal Issues

Amanda's partner and her parents commenced proceedings in negligence against the local area health service responsible for the psychiatric unit in which Amanda had been an inpatient. Phillip and Amanda's parents sought recovery of damages for psychiatric injury caused by her death. Phillip also claimed damages under the Compensation to Relatives Act 1987 (NSW) for his and Angus's loss of the pecuniary benefits Amanda would have provided had she survived.

The case against the local area health service was that Amanda was prescribed inappropriate medication. It was alleged that she should have been prescribed a more appropriate antidepressant than dothiepin, and at a higher dose. She had a major depression and the dose prescribed was almost homeopathic. Even if it were reasonable to prescribe dothiepin, it should have been increased to well beyond 75 mg daily, to therapeutic levels. She also should have been prescribed major tranquillisers such as olanzapine or quetiapine, to augment the antidepressant effects of dothiepin.

Finally, and crucially, it was alleged that Amanda should not have been granted unescorted day leave on 14 May 2012 given her mood and thoughts the previous evening. That entry was not reviewed by any doctor prior to her discharge. The nurse did not pass it on at the time of handover.

The plaintiffs relied on the opinions of three psychiatrists, including an expert in women's mental health. All three experts were critical of the medication prescribed by the psychiatric team, the failure to recognise the seriousness of Amanda's condition, and the decision to allow her unescorted leave on 14 May 2012.

The experts' opinion was that there is no time in a woman's life when she is more at risk of mental illness than in the postpartum period. The mental illness can range from a mild mood disorder to psychosis. As a result of the potential seriousness of the mental illness, aggressive treatment is required. Treatment in a mother–baby unit is preferable.

While some psychiatrists might support the prescription of dothiepin, the majority would have advocated the use of a selective serotonin reuptake inhibitor in Amanda's case. The dose of dothiepin was unlikely to remedy her depression. Her anxiety, agitation and insomnia also required stronger medication. As the doses prescribed were too low to effect change, Amanda's depression remained largely untreated throughout her admission. It was hardly surprising that she still had a suicidal intention over two weeks into her admission, and acted on this.

The defendant admitted it breached its duty of care by wrongly allowing Amanda to go on unescorted leave on 14 May 2012, through failures to communicate and attach significance to the history recorded by the nurse on the evening of 13 May 2012. It served no expert evidence supporting Amanda's management in the psychiatric unit from 29 April 2012. It served no evidence disputing causation. The only evidence served was in relation to the severity of any psychiatric condition suffered by Phillip and Amanda's parents.

A coronial inquest determined that Amanda's death was avoidable. The civil case settled at mediation. The court, so far as it concerned Angus's claim, approved the settlement.

Discussion

It may be accepted that predicting suicide is impossible. There are, however, a number of red flags to which psychiatric nursing and medical staff should attach significance. Although Amanda was diagnosed as suffering from a major depression, a number of these warning signs were ignored. During her admission, she expressly referred to suicide by travelling into a wilderness area and not returning. She expressly told staff she was apprehensive about leave. She informed staff that she had suicidal intent. These symptoms were not acted upon. They were not communicated to Amanda's psychiatrist or the psychiatric registrar. She was not interrogated further about what she intended to do when she entered a wilderness area.

The focus of treatment in Amanda's case, at least initially, was on her insomnia. It appeared that staff assumed she would get better once her sleep improved. They did not attach sufficient significance to the insomnia being one part of a more serious condition. While a person's mood may improve with better sleep, the underlying depression also needs active treatment. Amanda's dose of dothiepin was less than half the dose recommended to have a therapeutic effect.

Clinical Principles

Amanda's story highlights the importance in psychiatric cases of erring on the side of caution when assessing the risk of self-harm. Often patients will inform staff that they have no intention of harming themselves when they have already formulated a plan to end their lives. In Amanda's case, the opposite occurred. She volunteered suicidal thoughts, but these symptoms were ignored.

It seems obvious that a patient suffering from a major depressive illness should be assumed to be at high risk of self-harm so long as their condition is untreated or partially treated. There was no basis to downgrade Amanda's risk assessment and allow her unescorted leave while she was on ineffectual doses of an antidepressant and sedative.

The case also highlights the severity of postpartum depression and the heightened risk of mental illness in this period. It is possible that Amanda's treating psychiatrist was concerned about prescribed medication passing to Angus through breastfeeding. While this may be a legitimate concern, it should not lead to undertreatment of a mother's mental illness, as occurred in Amanda's case.

Finally, the case again underscores the importance of communications from nursing staff in the management of hospital patients. If nursing staff had effectively communicated Amanda's mental state to medical practitioners, it is unlikely she would have been granted unescorted leave.

RESTRAINT

History

Alana Blum gave birth to her third child, Stephen, at a regional hospital near Brisbane on 2 April 2010. Alana was 36 years of age at the time of Stephen's birth. There were no problems with the pregnancy or the vaginal delivery. There was, however, an important aspect to her history that was overlooked. Alana had chronic schizophrenia. Her schizophrenia had proved to be resistant to first-line antipsychotic medications. As a result, she was prescribed clozapine, which is usually reserved for patients with treatment-resistant schizophrenia. Alana did well on clozapine. She had no side effects and no acute psychotic episodes. In the past, she had had numerous admissions for acute psychotic episodes. She had not been an inpatient or suffered an acute psychosis for four years.

Alana's general practitioner, Dr Graeme Philpott, was aware of Alana's history of schizophrenia. When he referred Alana to the maternity unit at the hospital for management of her pregnancy, labour and delivery, he neglected to advise staff of Alana's history of schizophrenia and the treatment she received for it.

Nonetheless, Alana had previously been admitted to the psychiatric unit attached to the hospital. Accordingly, the maternity staff ought to have been aware of her psychiatric history and her treatment with clozapine. Unfortunately, there was no communication between the maternity unit and the psychiatric unit prior to Alana's admission to hospital on 2 April 2010 for delivery of her son.

After Stephen's delivery, maternity staff allowed Alana to self-administer her clozapine. They did not appreciate the importance of the medication to Alana's condition. As events turned out, she did not regularly take the clozapine.

Three days after delivery, Alana suffered an acute psychotic episode and fell into a catatonic state. Catatonia is a rare condition. It is a serious condition because people with catatonia cannot feed themselves or maintain hydration. Alana was seen by the psychiatric registrar and diagnosed as suffering from an acute relapse of her schizophrenia due to non-compliance in taking clozapine. She was transferred to the psychiatric unit attached to the hospital and scheduled as an involuntary patient.

During her admission to the psychiatric unit, Alana was observed to switch between agitated and catatonic states. She was not given intravenous fluids and it was unclear whether she was maintaining sufficient dietary intake.

On the evening of 10 April 2010, Alana switched into an agitated state and spent the whole night pacing up and down the corridor. Nursing staff recorded a history of persecutory auditory hallucinations. They contacted the psychiatric registrar, but no further orders were made. At some time in the early morning of 11 April 2010, Alana ingested a caustic substance. She had access to a cleaner's trolley that had been either left in the corridor or left in an unlocked services room. Alana became distressed and in pain. She tried to induce vomiting by putting her fingers down her throat. Her lips were swollen and she had superficial burns to the skin on her chest and neck with swelling of her oropharynx.

Medical staff in the psychiatric unit attempted to sedate her by administering olanzapine 5 mg intramuscularly. Her agitation did not resolve. A call was made for help. Four burly wardsmen arrived to assist nursing staff and the junior doctor attending. Alana was restrained in a prone position by the four wardsmen and given 10 mg olanzapine. She then suffered a cardiac arrest with consequent hypoxic-ischaemic brain damage. She died 14 days later as a result of her hypoxic ischaemic encephalopathy.

Legal Issues

Alana's death was the subject of a coronial inquest. Subsequently, Alana's husband, Leonard, commenced civil proceedings on behalf of himself and his three children under the local Lord Campbell's Act and for nervous shock. He sued the hospital and Alana's general practitioner, Dr Philpott.

The case against Dr Philpott was for failing to inform maternity staff of Alana's schizophrenia and its treatment with clozapine. Dr Philpott admitted that he breached his duty of care to Alana by failing to inform the maternity staff of these facts. He, however, disputed causation, on the basis that the maternity unit ought to have known of Alana's schizophrenia in any event through proper communication with the psychiatric arm of the hospital. He argued that the conduct of the maternity and psychiatric units was overwhelmingly the cause of Alana's death. In addition, he maintained that Alana suffered what was a well-recognised risk of childbirth for a schizophrenic, an acute exacerbation of the condition.

The case against the hospital was for the lack of communication between its maternity and psychiatric arms. Alana should not have been managed during and after delivery in ignorance of her history of schizophrenia and treatment with clozapine. It was also alleged that her acute psychotic episode was poorly managed, especially as she had catatonia. In addition, Leonard alleged that it was entirely inappropriate to restrain Alana in a prone position in her state.

The case against the defendants was supported by a number of psychiatrists, a gastroenterologist and an emergency physician. The same type of expert evidence was served by the defendants.

The expert psychiatric evidence relied on by Leonard was that, if the maternity unit had been aware of the schizophrenia, Alana would have been closely monitored in the postnatal period and would not have been permitted to self-administer clozapine. The failure to take her clozapine materially contributed to her acute psychotic state or at least the severity of her acute psychotic state. The evidence also indicated that Alana's acute psychosis should have been treated more aggressively, especially as she suffered from catatonia. Catatonia required aggressive treatment to ensure adequate hydration and food intake so as to prevent the massive energy depletion that may result. The gastroenterologist evidence agreed that Alana was allowed to become dehydrated and malnourished.

If the severity of Alana's condition had been appreciated, then she would have been appropriately supervised and managed and would never have been able to access cleaning fluid. Ingestion of the caustic substance caused acute oesophageal injury with severe pain and distress requiring restraint. Thus, if she did not ingest the caustic substance, she would never have required restraint in the way that occurred.

The psychiatric evidence for the defendants was to the effect that postpartum exacerbation of schizophrenia is a well-recognised and unpredictable event. There was nothing that staff could have done to avert the catastrophe even if they had been aware of the past history of schizophrenia and the need for clozapine. This opinion failed to address how Alana could have been allowed to gain access to a caustic substance if she was being properly supervised. It did not deal with the method of restraint in a prone position. It did not address the proven effectiveness of clozapine in treating Alana's condition or the result of missing doses of the drug in the high-risk period after birth.

During the inquest, there was a suggestion by a gastroenterologist and pathologist that Alana's oesophageal injuries were caused by the ingestion of toothpaste. This was an interesting theory given the lack of evidence of Alana's accessing excessive amounts of toothpaste. It eventually became common ground that she ingested a caustic substance, which led to pseudomembranous oesophagitis. The gastroenterology opinion led by the defendants was that Alana would have died in any event as a result of the ingestion of a caustic compound. There was no question that ingestion of a caustic compound would have led to significant morbidity, but there was no evidence that Alana had perforation of her oesophagus or mediastinitis. The gastroenterology evidence for the plaintiff disagreed with the fatalistic view of the defendant expert. In any event, the hospital was still responsible for Alana's death by allowing her to have access to cleaning solutions in an acute psychiatric ward.

There was also a dispute as to whether Alana suffered a fatal arrhythmia caused by a combination of the drugs she was taking in the context of dehydration and malnutrition. In the end, it did not matter. All factors were likely to have contributed. Hypoxia from a heavy-handed restraint with airway obstruction coupled with any dehydration or electrolyte disturbance and drug interactions from her acute psychosis caused the cardiac arrest and consequent brain damage.

The coroner found that Alana swallowed a caustic substance in the mental health unit, the precise identification of which was not possible. He found that the ingestion of the caustic substance caused intense pain and agitation resulting in vomiting. The ingestion did not directly cause death. But for the ingestion of the substance, the restraint would not have occurred.

The primary cause of death was positional asphyxia from the manner in which Alana was restrained. He found that there were a litany of failings by health professionals and the hospital, each compounding on the next stretching back to the time Alana was found to be pregnant and referred to the maternity unit of the hospital for management of the pregnancy, labour and delivery. The failings started with Dr Philpott's failure to communicate about the history of schizophrenia and included the failure to communicate adequately between maternity and psychiatric units of the hospital, the management of nursing staff in the maternity ward, the management of staff in the mental health unit, including the level of observation, and ultimately the failure to comply with essential precautions required in restraining someone in the prone position so as to avoid positional asphyxia.

The case settled at mediation and was approved by the Supreme Court.

Discussion

This case highlights in tragic circumstances the importance of basic communication between medical staff and nursing staff. Alana's postpartum management would have been markedly different if there had been proper psychiatric input into her management and awareness by maternity ward staff of her past history of schizophrenia and treatment with clozapine. Closer attention to her mental welfare would likely have taken place, although an acute exacerbation of her schizophrenia may not necessarily have been prevented.

It seems that, once medical staff were aware of the past history of schizophrenia, the seriousness of Alana's condition was not recognised and she was not managed appropriately. A consultant psychiatrist never reviewed Alana. No one thought to institute aggressive treatment, particularly in relation to electrolytes, fluid and oral intake even though she had catatonia. The lack of input from senior professionals and the absence of awareness of the risks of catatonia in acute psychotic conditions may represent a failing of training of junior psychiatric staff. There was a stupefying lack of response to Alana's clearly agitated state on the evening of 10 April 2010. She should not have been left alone pacing up and down the corridor with derogatory voices in her head.

It is frequently necessary to restrain patients for their own safety. Restraint should always involve the minimal amount necessary to achieve the desired purpose and must always bear in mind the risk of obstructing a patient's airway in the prone position.

Clinical Principles

Patients in an acute psychotic state are unable to look after themselves. The purpose of observations in an acute psychiatric unit is to ensure patients do not self-harm. This requires recognition of the seriousness of a patient's condition. There were a number of red flags in Alana's case that were ignored. It is disturbing to think that an acutely psychotic patient could access cleaning fluid on a trolley in what was thought to have been an appropriately managed unit.

Resuscitation of patients and restraint often involve the participation of a number of individuals. Proper restraint of a patient involves application of appropriate physical force and appreciation of the risk to the airway especially in vulnerable patients.

SYNCOPE

History

Willem Amundsen was born in 1982 and was generally well until he was 13 years old. One evening in 1995 he suddenly lost consciousness during dinner. He had no warning of impending collapse, and fell head first onto his plate. When he woke a couple of minutes later, he had no recollection of the event, and appeared well thereafter.

Willem's mother took him to their general practitioner, Dr Frank Morrow, for assessment. Dr Morrow noted that Mrs Amundsen had been diagnosed with temporal lobe epilepsy some years previously. Dr Morrow did not note any details of the symptoms experienced by Mrs Amundsen, and accepted the diagnosis of epilepsy without question. Dr Morrow referred Willem to a paediatric neurologist, who concluded that Willem had probably fainted, and he had not had a fit. The neurologist did not appear to consider any diagnosis other than fainting or fitting to account for Willem's syncope.

Two years later Willem consulted Dr Morrow following several weeks of light-headedness and a sensation of a dreamlike state. A sleep-deprived electroencephalogram thereafter revealed no epileptiform activity. Thus, it was not likely that Willem had epilepsy. It was not considered that Willem's symptoms may have been due to cerebral ischaemia due to reduced cardiac output associated with torsades de pointes.

When Willem was 17 he experienced headache which seemed to be associated with amine intolerance. He was treated with sumatriptan nasal spray, but this was not tolerated because of drowsiness and fatigue. He subsequently settled with pizotifen.

Willem then remained well until the following year, 2000, when he had a febrile illness and syncope. He lost consciousness for approximately 30 seconds, without warning, and was admitted to the local regional community hospital overnight under the care of Dr Morrow. The elder sister of Willem's girlfriend had glandular fever at the time, and Willem had serologic evidence consistent with current Epstein–Barr virus infection. Dr Morrow noted a pansystolic murmur, which had not been present previously.

The resident doctor at the local hospital recorded a history of lethargy and fever and the circumstances of Willem's syncope before admission. The night before, Willem had got up to get a drink of milk and suddenly collapsed. He had not got up quickly and had not experienced postural dizziness. Willem did not experience presyncope. Mr Amundsen caught Willem before he hit the floor. There was stiffening of his back, arms and legs, before he went limp. The resident doctor concluded that Willem had fainted.

Willem was discharged home, to use prochlorperazine as required for dizziness. He had a dystonic reaction and he was readmitted to the same hospital, later the same day. It was thought that the dystonic reaction was due to prochlorperazine, for which he was treated with benztropine. There was no further dystonia, and no further syncope in hospital. The systolic murmur persisted. He was discharged home three days after his second admission.

During the early hours of the morning following discharge from hospital, Willem had a cardiac arrest. Mr Amundsen found his son in bed, not breathing and without a pulse. Mr Amundsen commenced cardiopulmonary resuscitation and the ambulance was called. Willem had ventricular fibrillation from which was reverted to sinus rhythm by electrical cardioversion, and he was driven by ambulance to the local regional community hospital. He was then transferred by helicopter to a city teaching hospital.

An echocardiogram on arrival showed poor left ventricular contraction, with mitral regurgitation. The mitral valve was morphologically normal and it was felt that the mitral regurgitation was associated with left ventricular dysfunction. There was not dilation of the left atrium, suggesting that left ventricular dysfunction was of recent onset. There was transient prolongation of the QT interval, and left ventricular systolic function improved.

During his admission to the teaching hospital Willem experienced self-terminating torsades de pointes. Accordingly, the final diagnosis was long QT syndrome. Epstein-Barr virus infection had likely precipitated torsades de pointes and ventricular fibrillation.

Willem's convalescence was slow because of ischaemic brain damage. Subsequent investigations of Willem's family suggested that he had familial long QT syndrome. Mrs Amundsen had QT interval prolongation but Mr Amundsen did not. Willem's younger sister had evidence of a ventricular repolarisation abnormality with failure of the ECG to return to baseline before the next P wave. This repolarisation abnormality was probably due to long QT syndrome.

Legal Issues

Willem's family commenced legal proceedings against Dr Morrow, because he had failed to consider that Willem had Epstein-Barr virus myocarditis and did not refer Willem for cardiological review when he detected a new murmur in the context of documented Epstein-Barr virus infection.

Expert witnesses were consulted. The opinions of the defence experts were that cardiological review during the first admission to hospital was not required and that cardiac arrest could not have been anticipated. Expert witnesses for Willem considered that cardiological review was indicated, because of recurrent syncope, typical of torsades de pointes, and not typical of vasovagal syncope.

Expert witnesses for the defence opined that if a cardiologist considered the loss of consciousness was not due to a malignant arrhythmia, then continuous electrocardiographic monitoring would not have been required. However, these same experts accepted that if there was any doubt that syncope may have been due to a malignant arrhythmia, then continuous electrocardiographic monitoring was required.

Experts for the plaintiff considered that Willem had long QT syndrome. An expert witness general practitioner opined that cardiological review was required when Willem experienced syncope and had a pansystolic murmur which had not been detected previously. Syncope on all occasions should have been reviewed by a cardiologist.

The matter was not settled at mediation, and proceeded to trial in 2006. The trial judge found in favour of the plaintiff. An appeal by the defence in 2007 was unsuccessful.

Discussion

Willem's mother had been diagnosed with temporal lobe epilepsy, but she had not been screened for cardiac arrhythmias. Willem had experienced syncope in 1995, and a paediatric neurologist had suggested no further investigation at the time. Willem was not reviewed by a cardiologist following syncope in 1995.

This original description of sudden collapse without warning, and loss of consciousness for more than a minute was typical for a Stokes-Adams attack (sudden loss of cardiac output due to rapid ventricular tachyarrhythmia such as torsades de pointes, or complete heart block), and was not typical for vasovagal syncope (presyncope due to hypotension without compensatory tachycardia, collapse and prompt resumption of consciousness).

In 1997 Willem reported light-headedness and a dreamlike state. A sleep-deprived electroencephalogram was normal. Self-terminating torsades de pointes was not considered as a cause for presyncope. Again, Willem was not reviewed by a cardiologist.

When Willem presented in 2000 with a febrile illness and loss of consciousness for 30 seconds, recent exposure to glandular fever was noted and Epstein-Barr viral serology was requested. The cause of syncope was not further explored. The new onset pansystolic murmur was not investigated.

Although the description of Willem's sudden loss of consciousness without prodrome suggested torsades de pointes and did not suggest vasovagal syncope, it does not appear that a ventricular tachyarrhythmia was considered as the cause for loss of consciousness in 2000 (as it had not been considered in 1995).

This description suggested sudden loss of cardiac output resulting in seizure activity. The description was not typical of vasovagal syncope, in which the sufferer would usually experience presyncope and then slump, without stiffening of the limbs. The cause of syncope was not investigated further at the time.

If a cardiologist had been consulted following syncope in 1995 or in 2000 (or following presyncope in 1997 when epilepsy was excluded), it is likely that an arrhythmic aetiology for symptoms would have been considered. If a cardiologist had been consulted when Willem had Epstein-Barr virus infection and syncope, and a new pansystolic murmur, an echocardiogram would have been performed.

Irrespective of the result of the echocardiogram it is likely that a clinical diagnosis of viral myocarditis would have been made, and continuous electrocardiographic monitoring would have been performed pending resolution of Willem's illness.

The possibility of long QT syndrome and torsades de pointes would have been considered also. He would likely still have been monitored in hospital at the time of his cardiac arrest, and he would have been resuscitated promptly. The risk of neurological deficit would have been reduced, or eliminated.

If an echocardiogram had been performed during the first or second admission to hospital in 2000, it would likely have shown left ventricular dysfunction and mitral regurgitation, thereby strengthening the diagnosis of Epstein-Barr myocarditis.

Willem experienced dystonia after administration of prochlorperazine. Since the dystonia settled promptly following administration of benztropine, it is likely that dystonia was due to prochlorperazine, and not associated with long QT syndrome.

Although Willem had experienced syncope for 30 seconds prior to his first admission to the local hospital in 2000, and had a probable dystonic reaction to prochlorperazine, neither cardiological nor neurological review was requested before Willem was discharged home.

It is likely that if a cardiologist had been consulted, a diagnosis of Epstein-Barr virus myocarditis would have been made, and electrocardiographic monitoring would have been continued up to and beyond the time that Willem experienced cardiac arrest in ventricular fibrillation.

It is likely that if a neurologist had been consulted, a diagnosis of viral myocarditis also would have been made, and no further neurologic investigation would have been undertaken in respect of transient dystonia.

When Willem was transferred to the city teaching hospital there was initially poor left ventricular function, which improved. Accordingly, it is likely that transient left ventricular dysfunction was due more to hypoxia associated with cardiac arrest, than due to myocarditis. Nevertheless, the precipitating cause of ventricular fibrillation was likely Epstein-Barr viral infection and myocarditis. In retrospect, the period of syncope for 30 seconds prior to the first admission to the local hospital was probably due to self-terminating torsades de pointes.

Transient prolongation of QT interval following cardiac arrest raised the possibility that Willem had experienced torsades de pointes as a manifestation of long QT syndrome. Documented torsades de pointes confirmed the diagnosis.

Self-terminating torsades de pointes probably accounted for syncope as a teenager, but the paediatric neurologic opinion at the time was that Willem had simply fainted. Although Epstein-Barr virus infection probably precipitated ventricular fibrillation in 2000, this did not contradict the likelihood of torsades de pointes on previous occasions when Willem had experienced syncope or presyncope (in the absence of Epstein-Barr virus infection).

Clinical Principles

This case illustrates the importance of considering all potentially lethal causes of syncope. If neurological causes of syncope are excluded, or considered unlikely, then arrhythmic causes should be considered. If symptoms are not typical for vasovagal syncope, then other causes must be excluded.

Long QT syndrome may be associated with presyncope if torsades de pointes is self-terminating before the onset of syncope. Accordingly, it is important to consider long QT syndrome in an individual with presyncope, especially if there is a family history consistent with torsades de pointes.

VISUAL DISTURBANCE

History

Maria Stavros was born in 1961, and worked as a property developer. She was married to a general medical practitioner, Dr Yianni Stavros, with whom she had four children. Apart from a motor vehicle accident in 1990, Maria had been well until 2006.

On three occasions over several weeks in 2006, Maria experienced transient visual disturbances which caused her to stop driving each time the symptoms occurred. The visual disturbances resolved after a few minutes on each occasion, and she was able to continue driving. During the period when the visual disturbances occurred, she also experienced episodic light-headedness and a sensation of losing her footing.

Maria reported these symptoms to her husband, who was concerned that Maria may have experienced transient cerebral ischaemia, or had some other pathology to account for her symptoms. Neurological examination by Dr Stavros was unremarkable. Dr Stavros arranged a CT brain scan, transthoracic echocardiogram and cardiological review, with Dr Bernadette Ongley.

The radiologist reporting the brain scan noted the recent history of visual disturbances, and reported a probable lacunar infarct in the left basal ganglia. The echocardiogram showed a hypermobile atrial septum (atrial septal aneurysm) without evidence of a patent foramen ovale (PFO). Dr Stavros did not receive this report until 2013, when legal proceedings were underway. When Dr Stavros requested images from the 2006 study, they could not be found amongst Dr Ongley's archives.

When Dr Ongley reviewed Maria, she was aware of the result of the CT brain scan, but had not yet seen the report of the transthoracic echocardiogram. Dr Ongley noted the visual disturbances, light-headedness and losing her footing. Dr Ongley did not elicit a history of generalised visual disturbances or seeing squiggly lines. She requested further investigations to exclude a cardiac cause for the symptoms reported by Maria. The results of ambulatory blood pressure and electrocardiographic monitoring were unremarkable. Independently of Dr Ongley, Dr Stavros requested a magnetic resonance imaging (MRI) brain scan, and consultant neurological review.

Although the MRI images were affected by artefact, the consensus was that Maria had not had a stroke, and probably had an incidental finding of a hamartoma. The neurologist noted that Maria reported generalised visual disturbances which were not associated with headache, and that Maria had never experienced migraine. He also elicited a history of seeing squiggly lines at various sites in the visual fields. The neurologist did not note the history of light-headedness or of losing her footing.

The neurologist concluded that Maria's symptoms were migrainous in nature, but made the point that they were not due to migraine. Although he did not say as such at the time, it was his view in court later, that the episodes were not due to transient cerebral ischaemia. When Maria had been seen by the neurologist, she was reassured that her symptoms were benign and no further investigation was arranged by the neurologist.

Maria returned to Dr Ongley after the neurological review. She apologised to Dr Ongley that she may have been wasting Dr Ongley's time, since her brain was apparently normal. Dr Ongley indicated that a transoesophageal echocardiogram and bubble study were not required, since stroke had been excluded. Dr Ongley did not appear to have considered that Maria's symptoms may have been due to transient cerebral ischaemia.

The following year Maria experienced sudden onset of left hemiplegia, while attending to one of her children at home. She was transferred immediately by ambulance to the nearby city teaching hospital where there was CT scan evidence of cerebral infarction in the territory of the right middle cerebral artery. There was no major improvement with thrombolysis, and Maria was left with permanent disability, and was unable to resume paid work.

Following the stroke, a transoesophageal echocardiogram showed a PFO, as well as the atrial septal aneurysm. A thrombophilia screen was negative.

The PFO was closed percutaneously, and Maria experienced no further stroke. Following the stroke, Dr Ongley reviewed the initial transthoracic echocardiogram, and said to Dr Stavros that since the MRI brain scan the previous year had not suggested embolic stroke, transoesophageal echocardiographic assessment had not been indicated.

Legal Issues

Maria's family sued Dr Ongley for failure to investigate adequately cardiovascular causes for possible transient cerebral ischaemia in 2006. The matter went to trial.

Expert witnesses both for the defence and for the plaintiff agreed that hemiplegic stroke was likely the result of thromboembolism associated with Maria's PFO and atrial septal aneurysm. Expert witnesses for the defence and plaintiff also agreed that anticoagulation or closure of the PFO were appropriate treatment options to reduce the risk of subsequent stroke.

Expert witnesses for the defence maintained that the visual symptoms were migrainous in nature and that transoesophageal echocardiographic assessment was not indicated.

Expert witnesses for the plaintiff considered that Maria's presenting symptoms were probably due to transient cerebral ischaemia and that transoesophageal echocardiographic assessment was indicated.

Under detailed cross-examination by the defence barrister, the expert witnesses for the plaintiff agreed that transoesophageal echocardiographic assessment would have been indicated following recurrent episodes of visual disturbance while driving, even if those episodes were due to migraine. It was unclear in court exactly when each of the episodes of visual disturbance had occurred in relation to the first visit to Dr Ongley. However, given that the neurologist noted three previous episodes of visual disturbance soon after Maria had initially seen Dr Ongley, it was likely that Maria had in fact experienced three episodes of visual disturbance before she saw Dr Ongley.

The trial judge found in favour of the defence. The judge considered that the presenting symptoms were not likely to be due to transient cerebral ischaemia and that the assessments by Dr Ongley were adequate in the circumstances.

Discussion

Cardiologists are commonly consulted to consider cardiovascular causes for transient neurological symptoms. PFO and atrial septal aneurysm are more prevalent in patients with transient cerebral ischaemia or stroke than in the general population.

Dr Stavros was appropriately concerned that his wife may have experienced cerebral ischaemia associated with cardiac abnormalities, or may have had a structural brain lesion or epilepsy to account for her symptoms. Dr Ongley was appropriately concerned that Maria's symptoms may have been due to cardiovascular pathology. Dr Ongley considered that Maria's symptoms may have been due to changes in blood pressure, or transient AF, but did not appear to consider that the symptoms may have been due to transient cerebral ischaemia associated with PFO and atrial septal aneurysm.

At the time of initial review, Dr Ongley had not seen the transthoracic echocardiogram, and may not have been aware of the presence of an atrial septal aneurysm. At the time of subsequent review after the MRI scan, Dr Ongley accepted Maria's statement that she had not had a stroke. Neither migrainous symptoms nor possible transient cerebral ischaemia were mentioned at the time.

In this case the increased risk for stroke would have been highlighted if transoesophageal echocardiography and a bubble study had been requested in 2006, since such studies would likely have demonstrated a PFO. A transthoracic echocardiogram with a Valsalva manoeuvre (with or without bubbles) would have been an inferior alternative to transoesophageal assessment, because of the reduced spatial resolution of transthoracic examination compared with transoesophageal examination.

If Dr Ongley had proceeded with a transoesophageal echocardiographic study in 2006, the PFO would likely have been demonstrated, and anticoagulation or PFO closure would have been offered, to reduce the risk of stroke. These treatments would likely have been implemented irrespective of whether the original symptoms were thought to be due to transient cerebral ischaemia or otherwise. The risk for Maria having a disabling stroke would have been reduced (although perhaps not eliminated) by anticoagulation or PFO closure.

The fact that the MRI scan did not suggest a previous cerebral infarction did not contradict the history of transient neurological symptoms which may have been due to transient cerebral ischaemia without infarction.

Clinical Principles

When a patient presents with transient neurological symptoms, it is important to include amongst differential diagnoses to explain those symptoms any potentially serious diagnoses, unless and until those serious diagnoses are excluded and replaced with a benign diagnosis.

The precise history of transient neurological symptoms is often difficult to elucidate. In this case the histories recorded by Dr Ongley and the neurologist were not identical. Maria was interrogated by at least three medical practitioners. It is possible that her stated recollection of symptoms was influenced by the nature of questioning on each occasion. It is also possible that the various medical practitioners interpreted and recorded Maria's symptoms differently from what she recalled.

Sadly, none of the practitioners (Dr Stavros, Dr Ongley or the neurologist) spoke to each other at the time about Maria's symptoms or the need for further investigation. If they had spoken, it is likely that the possibility of transient ischaemia would have been discussed, and that the potential risk of the atrial septal aneurysm would have been recognised. Transoesophageal echocardiographic assessment including a bubble study would have been arranged. Then, the history of recurrent transient neurological symptoms, and the atrial septal aneurysm and the patient foramen ovale would all have been known. Dr and Mrs Stavros would likely have requested closure of the PFO, or anticoagulation.

THINGS MAY NOT BE AS THEY SEEM

History

Alice Tunbridge was a 49-year-old trained nurse who worked in a small private hospital on one side of a state border. She told the general practitioners in town that she had a complex anaemia that was managed by haematologists at a referral hospital on the other side of the border. Various doctors in the general practice who she attended in her home town treated her with oral and parenteral iron. She told her doctors from time to time that she had been admitted to hospital across the border for intravenous infusions.

Alice attended her general practice clinic on a total of 137 times over 17 years. Many of these attendances were for treatment of migraine headaches. She was prescribed narcotics at the clinic, often with take-home supplies of oxycodone suppositories.

The consultations occurred when computerised records were not routinely used in general practice clinics. Alice was happy to see any of the four doctors at the clinic and no single doctor seemed to have overall management of her condition. On several occasions Alice attended the practice to remove a cannula, which she said had been inserted during a recent hospitalisation.

Some months prior to her death one of the doctors at the clinic began to suspect that she may have been suffering from Munchausen syndrome. Nothing was done by the general practitioner at that time, and several weeks later Alice died suddenly.

A coronial inquest was ordered to determine the manner and cause of Alice's death. After making inquiries at the interstate hospital, no record was discovered of her ever attending the hospital over the border. There was an opinion expressed at the coronial inquiry that she may have been taking the oxycodone orally.

Legal Issues

The inquest resulted in finding that Alice died as a result of an overdose of oxycodone.

The coroner requested opinions from a general practitioner expert, neurologist and psychiatrist. Criticisms were levelled at the general practitioners who had seen Alice over 17 years. While the general practice clinic was in a difficult position as it had taken Alice's word about her conditions for many years, the expert evidence suggested that the general practitioners in the practice should have ensured that what she was claiming was in fact correct, especially as they never received any discharge summaries or correspondence from the interstate hospital or the haematologists.

The general practitioner expert was also critical of the management of Alice's migraines. These were treated by the administration of frequent doses of narcotics with take-home supplies without ever seeking the advice of a neurologist.

Alice's family is considering whether to instruct lawyers to investigate and prosecute civil proceedings in negligence against the treating general practitioners.

Discussion

"The Munchausen Syndrome is characterised by the tireless and repeated attempts, carried out by the affected individual, to obtain hospitalisation following an extremely credible and dramatic representation of physical symptoms. The condition was first described by Asher in 1951; the author saw fit to link the syndrome to the name of the Baron of Munchausen, the character described by Raspe, famous for the tendency to tell lies, thus highlighting what is the main element of the disease which is the tendency to lie to doctors about one's health, filling one's own life with dramatic events (pseudologia fantastica)." (1)

Patients with Munchausen syndrome are often extremely plausible and convincing, and sometimes able to fool even the most diligent of practitioners. It is unfortunate that the doctors in this case did not seek correspondence from the hospital about her supposed long-term anaemia management or the need for her repeated iron injections. Nor did they seek advice from a consultant about her persistent migraine.

The doctors should have suspected Munchausen syndrome every time Alice presented with an intravenous cannula, allegedly left in after an admission to hospital. The repeated prescription of opiates to treat migraine should have raised the possibility of addiction.

Alice was obviously a difficult patient who had deceived several doctors. The reliance on hand-written notes whose legibility may have been difficult for the different doctors to understand may have adversely affected communication. When Munchausen syndrome was eventually suspected, no effort was made to obtain expert assistance. Such assistance may have reduced the risk of self-harm associated with opiate use and intravenous cannulation.

When Munchausen syndrome is suspected, the possibility should be discussed with colleagues so that a management plan can be developed to reduce the risks of harm to the patient.

Alice was a trained nurse working locally and was probably well known to the general practitioners who cared for her. They would likely have had to interact with her at the local private hospital. The fact that she was a professional colleague further compounded the situation, as she would have been seen as a credible fellow professional.

Clinical Principles

Always be suspicious when a patient's history does not ring true. Patients may withhold important information for a variety of reasons. They may not remember something, they may be embarrassed about certain private details, they may be trying to manipulate the practitioner. Patient, probing history-taking is critical. So is being alert to the possibility of unusual conditions.

As in this case, always suspect Munchausen syndrome when the story doesn't make sense. The clinic doctors must have found it curious that they received no correspondence from the hospital across the border. They apparently made no attempt to obtain reports from the haematologists.

The diagnosis of migraine was accepted at face value. It would have been appropriate to request an expert opinion about management. A consultant neurologist may have suspected factitious disease and addiction. Early intervention may have averted Alice's untimely death.

References

1. Mayer, G., 2000. Facolt di Psicologia, Universita delgi Studi la Sapienza Roma Italia. Clin. Ter. 351–355.

HEADACHE

History

Beryl Austin was widowed and lived alone. For several years she had consulted Dr Abdul Azab (general practitioner) because of hypertension and hypercholesterolaemia, for which she was treated with ramipril and simvastatin. She did not smoke cigarettes.

In the autumn of 2009 Beryl, then aged 63 years, experienced chest pain while mopping the floor late in the afternoon. She called the ambulance and was transferred to the local regional hospital. She was haemodynamically stable (blood pressure 130/85 mmHg, pulse regular at 70/min). There was inferior ST elevation myocardial infarction (STEMI), for which she received thrombolytic therapy with an appropriate dose of tenecteplase.

She was not transferred to an interventional centre for coronary angiography, because it would have taken several hours to get there. Beryl remained free of chest pain following thrombolysis, and the ST segments returned to baseline. Since thrombolysis was effective, there was not an indication for urgent transfer to an interventional centre.

In addition to thrombolytic therapy, Beryl appropriately received aspirin, clopidogrel and heparin. She weighed 64 kg. A weight-adjusted bolus of heparin (5,000 U) was followed by an infusion (20 mL/hr × 50 U/mL = 1,000 U/hr) via a syringe pump. A separate syringe pump was used to infuse normal saline (166 mL/hr). While Beryl's gown was being changed by the nurses in the emergency department during the evening, the heparin and saline lines were inadvertently connected to the wrong infusion pumps. As a result, heparin 15,000–18,000 U was administered over three to four hours, rather than 8,000–9,000 U over that period, as was intended.

During the evening Beryl developed bruising and haematomas over her limbs and torso. When she was transferred to the intensive care unit around midnight, the medication error was recognised. The heparin infusion was suspended, approximately one hour later. At 02:15 h the APPT was >200 secs (>2.5 times the upper limit of the therapeutic range, therapeutic range of APPT on heparin 48–80 secs). An incident form was completed, noting the medication error, and the bruising and haematomas.

Beryl slept intermittently during the early hours of the morning until she experienced severe headache commencing around 05:00 h, and vomited old blood. The nurses noted that Beryl was clutching her head. She stopped complaining of headache following administration of morphine 5 mg intravenously, and appeared to be sleeping. The APPT at 06:30 h was 58 secs (i.e. still above the normal range, and still within the therapeutic range, more than five hours after the heparin infusion had been stopped). Neurologic observations were commenced.

At around 07:00 h the ward doctor noted the bruising and headache, and requested that blood be cross-matched. He did not consider any therapy to reduce bleeding, and did not request a brain scan.

It was not until several hours later that Beryl was reviewed by the daytime medical staff, who noted the medication error overnight. Beryl was now unrousable. The medical staff suspected intracerebral bleeding.

By the time a CT scan was performed there was extensive intracerebral bleeding and Beryl passed away soon after.

Legal Issues

The medication error was recognised by the hospital staff. An incident form was completed and the case was reviewed within the hospital, after Beryl's death. It was concluded that intracerebral bleeding was due to tenecteplase and not due to heparin. It was considered by the hospital that the dose of tenecteplase was appropriate and that the overdose of heparin did not contribute to cerebral haemorrhage (i.e. there was no blame attributable to the hospital staff who had caused the heparin overdosage).

Beryl's family commenced proceedings against the hospital, because her death due to cerebral bleeding was avoidable if she had not received an overdose of heparin.

Expert witnesses for Beryl's family and for the hospital were consulted. There was disagreement between the experts as to the timing and quantum of heparin overdosage, and there was disagreement about the contribution of heparin overdosage to intracerebral bleeding. There was also disagreement about the need for neurologic observations. Whereas the plaintiff's expert considered that close neurologic monitoring (and medical review) was mandatory, the defence expert opined that, "intensive or frequent monitoring could have disturbed the patient more and would not have helped in management". The matter was settled at mediation in 2013, four years after Beryl's death.

Discussion

When Beryl presented with exertional chest pain she was initially managed appropriately for an acute coronary syndrome. When there was evidence of STEMI Beryl received thrombolytic therapy, since cardiac catheterisation was not available at the local regional hospital, and transfer to an interventional centre would have taken several hours.

Administration of aspirin, clopidogrel and heparin was all according to contemporary guidelines. When Beryl's gown was being changed, it is likely that both of the intravenous lines were disconnected simultaneously from their respective infusion pumps. Insufficient care was taken to ensure that each line was reconnected to the correct pump. Alternatively, the infusion rates of each pump were programmed incorrectly.

If the heparin infusion had been stopped immediately the error was identified, the incremental anticoagulant effect of further additional heparin would have been eliminated. As it was, the heparin infusion was not suspended until approximately one hour after the error was noted, and the APTT was not measured until approximately two hours after the error was noted.

An appropriate course would have been to stop the heparin infusion immediately the error was detected, to document forthwith the APTT, and to seek expert medical advice without delay. This would have reduced the ongoing risk of anticoagulation overdose, and would have highlighted the option to reverse or partially reverse the anticoagulant effect of heparin. Reversal of the anticoagulant effect of heparin at this time would have afforded Beryl the best chance of avoiding ongoing bleeding complications.

By the time the medication error was noted, Beryl had received approximately twice the intended dose of heparin over a period of three to four hours. Although the presence of extensive bruising was observed and recorded after the medication error was detected, the anticoagulant effect of heparin was not antagonised with protamine. There was no evidence that those caring for Beryl had considered at the time the risks and benefits of reversing heparin with protamine.

If the anticoagulant effect of heparin was reversed or partially reversed with protamine, the risk of bleeding generally, and intracerebral bleeding in particular, would have been reduced. Although it could have been argued that reversing the effect of heparin may have increased the risk of further coronary thrombosis, this was not a reason to ignore the option of reversing the heparin. There was a strong indication to consult immediately with cardiology and haematology experts during the night to ensure that the risks and benefits of various management options were adequately considered.

In this case it was vital to weigh the ongoing bleeding risk of unreversed anticoagulation in the presence of extensive cutaneous bruising and haematomas against the potential coronary arterial thrombotic risk of reversing anticoagulation. These considerations should have been documented in the clinical notes at the time of consideration, so that subsequent carers would be aware of the previous considerations.

Given that Beryl had inferior ST elevation initially, it was likely that there had been occlusion of the right or circumflex artery, and not occlusion of the left anterior descending artery. Hence the morbid risk of possible intracerebral bleeding was likely greater than the morbid risk of recurrent thrombosis of the infarct-related artery.

When Beryl experienced severe headache and was clutching her head, and vomited old blood, neurologic observations were commenced (either because of suspected intracerebral bleeding, or because of the recognised risk of intracerebral bleeding). The sudden onset of severe headache, sufficient to warrant intravenous morphine and neurological monitoring, in the context of heparin overdosage and extensive bruising, meant the likely presence of intracranial bleeding. Immediate medical review was mandated.

At the time of the initial medical review, the ward doctor requested that blood be cross-matched. The anticoagulant effect of heparin was not reversed with protamine, and specialist physicians were not consulted.

It was appropriate to assume that the risk of intracranial haemorrhage was higher than usual when there was extensive bruising and haematomas, and haematemesis, in the context of heparin overdosage. It appears that the urgency of the situation was ignored when Beryl appeared asleep after intravenous morphine. By the time Beryl was reviewed by medical staff later in the morning, she was unconscious because of irreversible brain damage, and the opportunity to reverse the anticoagulation effect of heparin had been lost.

Clinical Principles

This case illustrates the need to ensure the correct connection of intravenous lines to infusion pumps. It is standard nursing practice when administering intravenous medication for two qualified individuals to check the dose (and the name of the medication and the expiry date). Accordingly, two qualified individuals should have checked the intravenous lines when they were reconnected to the pumps. There is no evidence that this was done.

This case also illustrates the need to consider immediately the risks of a medication error. As soon as the nursing staff recognised that there had been inadvertent excessive administration of heparin, they should have sought expert medical advice. Completion of an incident form was not a substitute for urgent advice.

The need to consider the downstream risks of the medication error was emphasised when there was already evidence of bleeding complications (extensive cutaneous bruising and haematomas). It was not appropriate to wait until there was headache, likely due to intracranial haemorrhage, before seeking medical advice.

Contrary to the opinion of the defence expert, close neurological monitoring was mandatory when intracranial haemorrhage was suspected, because of the morbid risk associated with ongoing cerebral haemorrhage.

The local regional hospital review of the events appeared biased. The reviewers played down the possible or likely role of heparin overdosage in intracranial bleeding and death. In this case impartial review by a third party unrelated to the hospital was required.

MECHANISM OF STROKE

History

On 20 August 2005, Suzana Lazarevic, a 53-year-old real estate agent, fell down some stairs at a property she was showing to potential purchasers. She injured her left ankle. Although she thought it was a sprain, she decided to consult her general practitioner, Dr David Ewart, just in case it was more serious. She consulted him on the same day. He ordered an x-ray of Suzana's left foot and ankle, which revealed a fracture of the calcaneus and a calcaneocuboid dislocation. Dr Ewart thought it was a minor fracture and told Suzana that she had "a chip" in one of the bones in her foot. He referred Suzana to a physiotherapist, Mr Cam Lucas, for further treatment of the fracture. He applied a plaster of Paris back slab and advised Suzana to use crutches and not to weight-bear for six weeks.

Four weeks after the injury, Suzana developed pain in the left calf. She also had swelling of the left foot and ankle. She told Mr Lucas about the pain. She mentioned that she had lost her footing in the bathroom and might have strained a muscle. On examination, there was tenderness of the calf muscle belly. Mr Lucas diagnosed a muscle strain and applied interferential ultrasound.

Suzana also returned to see Dr Ewart because of the left calf pain. He made a provisional diagnosis of a muscular tear and referred her back to Mr Lucas for further treatment. Mr Lucas continued to treat Suzana with pulsed ultrasound therapy, interferential therapy and the use of compression bandages.

On 10 October 2005, Suzana was awakened by a severe headache. It was the worst headache she had ever experienced. She could not localise it to any particular region. It had not been present when she went to bed, and it had not awakened her earlier in the night. She complained to her husband about the headache and he decided to drive her quickly to the local hospital emergency department.

At the local hospital, Suzana recounted the history of being awakened suddenly with a severe headache. She also told staff about the recent fracture of the left foot and ankle, and the recent onset of left calf pain. She had no other symptoms and, on examination, no neurological deficits. Emergency staff considered a subarachnoid haemorrhage (SAH) as the provisional working diagnosis and ordered an urgent computed tomogram (CT) scan without contrast of the brain. The CT scan showed no abnormality. Susana was kept in for overnight observation under the care of the neurology team.

Overnight from 10 to 11 October 2005, Suzana developed left-sided weakness and visual field loss. These abnormalities were identified by nursing staff on the morning of 11 October 2005. Suzana was transferred to the area's tertiary referral hospital.

At the tertiary referral hospital, Suzana underwent an MRI brain scan with magnetic resonance angiography (MRA). This demonstrated a right-sided cerebral infarction. She was told she had suffered a thromboembolic stroke. The neurology team then ordered a battery of tests to identify the source of the clot. Although she had a past history of palpitations, there was no evidence of any clot within the heart on transthoracic echocardiography. There had never been a formal diagnosis of AF. The transthoracic echocardiogram, however, suggested the existence of a patent foramen ovale (PFO).

Cerebral angiography did not identify any site of narrowing. Because of the antecedent left calf pain, Suzana underwent a duplex scan of her calves, which failed to demonstrate any deep venous thrombosis (DVT). Suzana was commenced on aspirin and heparin. The working diagnosis was a paradoxical stroke from a DVT in the calf going through the PFO and lodging in the posterior cerebral arterial circulation. Suzana made reasonable progress with rehabilitation, but was left with a permanent visual field loss and left-sided weakness mainly affecting her left leg. After discharge from hospital, the PFO was eventually closed.

Legal Issues

Suzana commenced proceedings against Dr Ewart, Mr Lucas and the local hospital. She retained a number of lawyers over the years, each giving conflicting advice about her prospects and which party was to blame. In the end, she believed that all were responsible and kept them all in the claim.

The case against Dr Ewart was that he failed to appreciate the severity of the initial injury and that he failed to consider the possibility of a DVT when Suzana developed left calf pain four weeks into immobilisation. There was a conflict between the expert general practitioner evidence served by Suzana and Dr Ewart in relation to referral to an orthopaedic surgeon for management of her fracture-dislocation. The argument was that with referral, an orthopaedic surgeon would have been more likely to suspect DVT when left calf pain and swelling developed. A duplex scan of the left calf would have confirmed DVT, Suzana would have received anticoagulant therapy, and subsequent stroke would have been avoided. There was agreement between the experts in relation to the need for Dr Ewart to have suspected a DVT when Suzana developed left calf pain and swelling. Both agreed that duplex scanning ought to have been ordered. Neither could express a firm view about whether the investigation would have revealed a DVT. That question was to be determined by vascular surgeons and vascular physicians.

Similar allegations were made against Mr Lucas for failing to consider the possibility of DVT in the context of prolonged lower limb immobilisation and the sudden onset of calf pain. In addition, the plaintiff's physiotherapist expert said that interferential ultrasound carries a risk of embolisation from a DVT and is contraindicated until such time as a DVT had been excluded. Ultimately, the dispute between the physiotherapy experts was whether referral for duplex scanning or referral back to Dr Ewart for consideration of duplex scanning would have led to the diagnosis of a DVT, anticoagulant therapy and avoidance of the paradoxical stroke.

The case against the hospital was that it ought to have worked out that Suzana had had a thromboembolic stroke and administered thrombolysis shortly after her presentation to the emergency department with the sudden onset of a severe headache. The case against the local hospital was supported by an emergency specialist but not a neurologist. The hospital relied on the opinions of neurologists. There was a dispute in relation to causation.

Given the sudden onset of a severe, 'thunderclap' headache, it was agreed among the experts that SAH was at the top of the list of differential diagnoses. Other diagnoses included a thromboembolic stroke, neoplasia and infection. All agreed that a CT scan without contrast was a reasonable screening test to confirm or exclude SAH. Once a SAH had been excluded, then a diagnostic work-up ought to have ensued to confirm or exclude an ischaemic stroke or other intracranial pathology. That entailed an MRI/MRA scan or a CT scan with contrast, a CT angiogram or cerebral angiography. It was also considered that a lumbar puncture was appropriate.

Suzana, however, had been told that whatever the result of a lumbar puncture, she would need angiography to ascertain if there was a cerebral aneurysm that required clipping or coiling. She therefore refused to undergo a lumbar puncture, but agreed to angiography. CT angiography was ordered for the next day. The CT angiography could only occur at the tertiary referral hospital. Suzana's expert was of the opinion that urgent transfer to the tertiary hospital should therefore have occurred that evening.

There was a dispute among the vascular surgical experts as to whether Suzana had a DVT of her left leg. It was agreed that her symptoms in the context of four weeks of immobilisation were highly suggestive of a left calf DVT. The duplex study at the tertiary hospital failed to identify a DVT. The expert vascular surgeons accepted that duplex scans have a false negative rate. They also thought it possible that there was a small DVT that had broken off completely, travelled via the inferior vena cava to the right atrium, across the PFO into the left atrium and thence via the left ventricle and aorta to the brain, to cause the stroke.

It was argued by the defendants' vascular surgeon that, if there had been a DVT, the clot would have passed from the left calf veins preferentially into the pulmonary circulation rather than through the PFO. A PFO is not open at all times. For the PFO to be open so as to permit a clot to pass through it, pressure in the right atrium must be higher than pressure in the left atrium. This may occur with coughing or straining, or if the right heart pressures are elevated because of pulmonary emboli.

The plaintiff could not prove that there was any reason for there to be a sudden increase in pulmonary blood pressure. While the clinical records described some chest pain, the lung perfusion ventilation scan did not reveal pulmonary embolism. Because of a negative ventilation perfusion scan performed at the tertiary hospital, there was no pulmonary embolism and, by inference, no DVT.

A number of cardiologists gave evidence about an alternative source of the thrombus. It was suggested that, because of the history of palpitations, Suzana had AF, making it likely that she had a cardiac thrombus. The dispute was somewhat arid in that the treating physicians at the tertiary hospital concluded that Suzana had had a paradoxical stroke. Moreover, Suzana did not have a history of AF, but had a past history of intermittent palpitations due to mechanisms other than AF. These had been extensively investigated by a cardiologist, who diagnosed her with left atrial ectopic beats and trivial mitral incompetence.

In the end, the dispute between the cardiac thrombosis theory and the DVT theory and paradoxical stroke became secondary to whether there had been an unreasonable delay in transferring Suzana to the tertiary hospital for CT angiography, an MRI/MRA scan, or cerebral angiography, and in consequence a failure in instigating thrombolysis. The origin of the clot did not matter to the institution of thrombolytic treatment.

There was no question that it was reasonable for the local emergency department to consider SAH as a working diagnosis. Suzana presented with classic symptoms of SAH. It was reasonable to perform a noncontrast CT scan as well as to recommend a lumbar puncture. Suzana refused to undergo a lumbar puncture because she wanted to proceed straight to CT angiography.

In order to succeed in her claim, Suzana needed to have had a diagnosis of a thromboembolic stroke within about 4.5 hours of the onset of symptoms of stroke (or earlier in the opinion of some neurologists). For this to have occurred, the SAH needed to have been excluded, and a provisional diagnosis of a thromboembolic stroke made. Suzana could then have been transferred to the tertiary hospital within time so as to undergo CT angiography as a precursor to the prescription of thrombolysis. Suzana was thus confronted by a difficult onus in proving what would have happened but for the hospital's alleged breach in failing to consider a thromboembolic stroke. The hurdle was too high. Suzana could only establish that it was possible rather than probable that she would have undergone thrombolysis within 4.5 hours. This is because she was unlikely to have sufficient neurological signs (or progression) at the time of transfer. She only developed neurological symptoms (rather than headache) overnight from 10 to 11 October 2005. The headache had resolved with analgesia.

Suzana's claim was high risk and, in the end, speculative in relation to causation. Unfortunately, early on in the investigation of a claim, she was advised that she had a "straightforward" claim for failing to receive "clot busting" medication early enough. This uninformed opinion made it difficult to extricate Suzana from the medicolegal mire she found herself in.

Proceedings were dismissed.

Discussion

To succeed in a medical negligence case a plaintiff needs to prove not only breach of a duty of care, but also causation in the sense that the breach of duty was a necessary condition for the suffering of the alleged harm. In this case, Suzana was able to establish that Dr Ewart and Mr Lucas breached their duty of care to her by not considering she had a left calf DVT. She could not establish that an earlier duplex scan would have led to diagnosis of a DVT. She had difficulty in proving that she had even suffered a paradoxical stroke.

Even if she established an unreasonable delay in considering and excluding a thromboembolic stroke, she was unlikely to succeed against the local hospital for that failure because of the uncertainty in establishing that thrombolysis treatment could have been commenced within an appropriate timeframe or that it would have been effective in preventing her permanent neurological deficits.

The subject of thrombolysis treatment for stroke is frequently raised in medicolegal litigation. It is inaccurate and glib to suggest to a patient that she would have had a significantly better outcome with early thrombolytic treatment or that there are no impediments to the prompt administration of thrombolysis. While dedicated stroke units seek a "door to needle" interval of one hour, this is unlikely to be realistic in the majority of emergency departments, particularly in regional centres.

This case highlights the frequent debate between when it becomes too late to commence thrombolytic therapy or if permanent deficits can be prevented. There is often confusion about the time of onset of a stroke and what is meant by a "wake up stroke".

A "wake up stroke" is regarded as a situation where a patient wakes up with symptoms of stroke (1). Whether headache is a symptom of a thromboembolic stroke is often a subject of debate, as it was in Suzana's case. Expert neurologists relied on by the hospital considered Suzana to have had a wake up stroke because she woke up with a headache and her headache was a symptom of the stroke. The countervailing argument was that the stroke had its onset overnight from 10 to 11 October 2005 with the development at an unspecified time of visual field loss and left-sided weakness. Headache does not necessarily represent brain parenchymal damage. The negative CT scan without contrast may have been evidence that the cerebral infarction had not occurred with the headache.

The time window for the administration of thrombolytic therapy to reverse or minimise the effects of stroke is 4.5 hours from the time of onset of the stroke. If headache was a symptom of the stroke, then thrombolysis would never have been initiated in Suzana's case. She plainly could not receive it until SAH had reasonably been excluded. If Suzana had agreed to a lumbar puncture, then that also was a relative contraindication to the administration of thrombolysis. Headache may occur in the context of an ischaemic stroke relating to injury to a vessel wall, but not to injury to brain parenchyma.

The likelihood and degree of recovery from a stroke relates to the National Institutes of Health Stroke Scale Score at the time of administration of thrombolysis and the time at which thrombolysis is given in relation to the time of onset of the stroke (2).

According to the Clinical Guidelines for Stroke Management 2010 by the National Stroke Foundation, intravenous thrombolysis should be given as early as possible in carefully selected patients with acute ischaemic stroke as the effect of thrombolysis is time-dependent. The recommendations are for therapy to commence in the first few hours, but may be used up to 4.5 hours after stroke onset.

While it is reasonable to have guidelines for best clinical practice, this does not mean that every failure to adhere to a guideline is negligent. There are often mitigating factors and practical considerations that mean hard-and-fast rules are impractical.

The case also highlights the failure to apply common sense and logic to medical problems. While it was possible that Suzana had torn her calf muscle, this could not be assumed to have been the case without first ruling out serious pathology such as a DVT. If Dr Ewart or Mr Lucas had ordered the investigation, then a lot of uncertainty would have been avoided. There may well have been different medical and legal outcomes.

Clinical Principles

Strokes may be ischaemic or haemorrhagic. It is important to exclude both as quickly as possible. A CT scan without contrast is a reasonable screening test for SAH, but should not be the end point of investigation. A negative CT scan without contrast is not an excuse to take the foot off the pedal of a diagnostic work up. Time may still be of the essence for other differential diagnoses. In many cases, the utility of a screening test is overstated. For example, if a patient presents to an emergency department with the sudden onset of a severe headache, a negative CT scan without contrast should not immediately lead to consideration of a nonorganic illness or the abandonment of timely investigations.

References

1. Rimmele, D.L., Thomalla, G., 2014. Wake up stroke: clinical characteristics, imaging findings and treatment option – an update. Frontiers in Neurology (Stroke) 5.
2. Lees, K.R., et al., 2010. Time to treatment with intravenous alteplase and outcome in stroke: an updated pooled analysis of ECASS, ATLANTIS, NINDS and EPITHET trials. Lancet 375, 1695–1703.

A PHARMACOLOGICAL NIGHTMARE

HISTORY

Trudy Mawson was in her early twenties when her doctor referred her to a rapid opioid detoxification clinic because of her heroin addiction. The clinic was run by Mr Bill Gladstone, who had studied psychology but was not qualified to practise as a psychologist. Mr Gladstone employed nurses and doctors at the clinic to administer and oversee the detoxification process, and to determine whether patients were medically fit to undergo treatment. One of the doctors employed was a recent overseas medical graduate, Dr Timothy O'Toole.

Trudy's doctor had attempted to manage her by gradual reduction of her narcotics, without success. He counselled her about the wisdom or otherwise of taking the step of rapid opioid detoxification. Trudy, having recently become a mother, was firm in her resolve to proceed with rapid detoxification. She was fed up with the methadone program.

On the day prior to the detoxification, Trudy had an electrocardiogram (ECG) that demonstrated a prolonged QT interval. This indicated an increased risk of malignant cardiac tachyarrhythmias, especially in the context of administration of drugs which may prolong the QT interval.

Trudy was admitted to the clinic from 08:00 h to 16:40 h for rapid detoxification. She signed a consent form which acknowledged that the use of naltrexone (which may be associated with torsades de pointes) was experimental and that naltrexone was of unproven therapeutic benefit. She also paid several thousands of dollars up-front for which she would receive no reimbursement.

Trudy reported that she had used heroin for four years and had been on the methadone program for five months. Both may cause QT prolongation and torsades de pointes. She admitted to taking heroin 0.2 g the day prior to admission for detoxification. It was noted that Trudy had no other comorbidity. The only recorded findings were those of a pulse rate of 101 bpm and a blood pressure of 123/90 mmHg. The ECG results were noted. Both methadone and benzodiazepines (which also may cause QT prolongation and torsades de pointes) were detected in her urine. These were not quantitated.

At 09:15 h Trudy was administered oral baclofen, butylscopolamine, clonidine, dexamethasone, flunitrazepam, indomethacin, subcutaneous octreotide (which may cause QT prolongation and torsades de pointes) and intramuscular diazepam and midazolam. At 10:30 h she received intramuscular metoclopramide (another potential cause of QT prolongation and torsades de pointes). At 11:30 h she was given oral metoclopramide.

During the day Trudy was given oral cephalexin and paracetamol, intramuscular diazepam and intravenous metoclopramide.

At ~12:00 h Trudy slipped over while going to the toilet. Slow release naltrexone was implanted at 13:30 h by Dr O'Toole. Lignocaine with adrenaline (further causes of QT prolongation and torsades de pointes) was used to anaesthetise the skin. At 17:00 h dexamethasone, octreotide and naltrexone were administered. Dr O'Toole left the clinic to go home before the treatment had finished.

There were no facilities at the clinic for remote monitoring of pulse or breathing.

At ~17:20 h a nurse observed that Trudy was not breathing. About ten minutes later the nurse was unable to detect a pulse. Cardiopulmonary resuscitation (CPR) was commenced, supplemental oxygen was given and an ambulance was called.

The ambulance arrived at 17:40 h and CPR was continued until Trudy was transferred to a major hospital where she was admitted at 18:24 h. Although there was return of spontaneous circulation, Trudy had irreversible brain damage and multiorgan failure, and died eight weeks later.

The cause of death was recorded as, "Hypoxic brain injury due to cardiorespiratory arrest due to cardiac arrhythmia or prolonged apnoea due to medical administration of sedatives or opioid antagonists".

LEGAL ISSUES

The matter was referred to the state coroner to determine the manner and cause of death. The potential for drugs to cause or exacerbate QT interval prolongation and precipitate malignant tachyarrhythmias was considered. Mr Gladstone had adopted a detoxification protocol without scientific merit and provided inadequate medical and nursing supervision at his clinic. Cardiopulmonary resuscitation was not commenced until approximately ten minutes after respiratory arrest was recognised.

Expert witnesses agreed that Trudy had QT prolongation. A defence expert opined that Trudy may have died anyway because of underlying long QT syndrome. A plaintiff expert considered that the combination of drugs administered at the clinic exacerbated long QT syndrome and caused cardiac arrest.

The coroner learned that two other patients had died previously after receiving drugs at Mr Gladstone's clinic.

Mr Gladstone was banned from offering mental health services, including counselling or related community health and welfare services.

Trudy's grandmother sued Dr O'Toole on behalf of Trudy's baby daughter under the local Lord Campbell's Act for the loss of financial and domestic support.

No expert evidence was served to support Dr O'Toole's assessment of Trudy's suitability for rapid opioid detoxification or his supervision of the process. He should not have certified her as safe for the treatment. He should have referred her to a cardiologist. He should have stayed around until the treatment was over rather than let the nursing staff deal with any emergency. There was a contest between experts as to whether Trudy would have been able to overcome her addiction, become gainfully employed and provide consistent domestic and childcare services for her daughter if she had not undergone rapid opioid detoxification. The civil case was settled at mediation. Mr Gladstone was not sued because he and his clinic were uninsured.

Discussion

Trudy was a vulnerable individual who was exposed to unethical behaviour by an unscrupulous individual. Mr Gladstone employed a recent medical graduate to implant naltrexone. Nurses were employed to administer oral, subcutaneous, intramuscular and intravenous drugs. If the staff at Mr Gladstone's clinic had recognised the prognostic importance of QT prolongation, Trudy could have avoided all the consequences of her inappropriate treatment.

The nurses at the clinic were slow to provide cardiopulmonary resuscitation after Trudy stopped breathing. Respiratory arrest was likely to have been a consequence of cardiac arrest due to a malignant ventricular tachyarrhythmia. If Trudy had been resuscitated promptly after the onset of respiratory arrest her chances of survival without hypoxic brain damage and multiorgan failure would have been higher.

Various Australian medical professional bodies have published guidelines for administration of sedation, including minimal standards for monitoring sedated patients. Mr Gladstone ignored all these.

Trudy had documented QT interval prolongation before admission to Mr Gladstone's clinic. Yet she received a miscellany of drugs which were known to cause QT prolongation and would increase the risk that Trudy would suffer a malignant ventricular arrhythmia.

In addition to the risks of QT prolongation from some of the drugs Trudy received, there are the issues such as sedation, respiratory depression, drug metabolism and half-life. If a drug is metabolised at a fixed rate, one half of the initial dose is active one half-life later, and a half of that amount is active another half-life later.

Diazepam has a half-life of 20–40 hours. The first dose of 5 mg was given at 09:15 h; another 5 mg was given at 10:40 h and a further 5 mg at 12:30 h. Thus, at 17:40 h there would have been 2.5 times the original dose in Trudy's system. The half-life of flunitrazepam is 20–30 hours. Approximately 80% of the morning dose would have remained active at 17:40 h.

Both metoclopramide and midazolam are sedative and can affect cardiac conduction. Octreotide may be associated not only with QT prolongation, but also with bradycardia. The manufacturers of naltrexone warn that it should be used with caution in patients receiving medications with potential adverse cardiovascular effects. Both lignocaine and adrenaline may be proarrhythmic.

It cannot be known exactly what drug or combination of drugs caused Trudy's cardiac arrest. What is known is that Trudy had not experienced symptoms to suggest a malignant arrhythmia before she attended Mr Gladstone's clinic. She did have QT interval prolongation the day before she received rapid opioid detoxification. Trudy experienced cardiac arrest after receiving several drugs known to cause QT prolongation and torsades de pointes. The combination of drugs used, the absence of monitoring and the delayed implementation of effective CPR were lethal.

There is an important principle of medical responsibility here. Dr O'Toole took instructions from an unqualified psychologist to prescribe and administer medications. Mr Gladstone's protocol for rapid opioid detoxification fell outside contemporary standards of practice. As a medical practitioner, Dr O'Toole's responsibility to his patients was not to do as he was told (by a licensed psychologist), but to determine independently whether proposed treatment was safe. He should have recognised that the rapid opioid detoxification protocol was reckless and potentially harmful, and he should not have chosen to be a part of it. He certainly should not have advised Trudy that she was safe to undergo the treatment when he knew she had a prolonged QT interval. She needed cardiology review and not a cocktail of drugs prescribed by an inexperienced doctor at the behest of an allied health professional.

Clinical Principles

Patients and doctors should consider carefully the risks and benefits of expensive therapies without proven benefit. Doctors need to carry out their own research on proposed treatments. Drug interactions are responsible for many serious illnesses. Do not guess that the prescription of multiple drugs will be safe. Check that they will be especially in the presence of a pre-existing medical condition.

QT interval prolongation is a red flag and should not be ignored, particularly if drugs known to cause QT prolongation and torsades de pointes are to be employed.

Guidelines for management of sedation exist to reduce the risks to patients. Staff caring for sedated patients must be skilled in recognition and prompt treatment of complications of sedation.

STEROID TOXICITY

History

John Wivell, aged 44, had a strong family history of atopy. He had had severe eczema since childhood, and recently had acne and conjunctivitis. John was a qualified tradesman, whose occupation since the age of 15 involved working in a very dusty environment. Over many years, John's general practitioner, Dr Martin Roberts, provided him with prescriptions for steroid and antibiotic eye drops, potent steroid creams and ointments to be applied to the skin including the face, and oral steroids. At various times he also took oral doxycycline and nonsteroidal skin preparations.

Dr Roberts referred John to a consultant dermatologist for continuing care. The dermatologist gave advice about the management of his severe skin disorder, including the use of moisturising preparations, oral antibiotics, steroid creams and ointments. He advised Dr Roberts to avoid prescribing potent steroids for the face.

The dermatologist's diagnoses were severe atopic dermatitis and severe steroid rosacea. Prominent areas of facial telangiectasia indicated irreversible changes because of chronic potent steroid use. He advised pimecrolimus cream as an alternative to local steroids, and strongly advised the use of dust mite covers for his bedding.

Two years later John was reviewed by the dermatologist, who confirmed his advice to use the same approach as previously, and reiterated his advice concerning facial steroids.

After a further two years the dermatologist performed RAST (radioallergosorbent) testing that demonstrated a high positive response to house dust mite, grass pollens and malassezia (fungus). He referred John to an immunologist to consider desensitisation to the identified allergens. If this approach did not achieve a degree of success, the dermatologist considered the next option would probably be an immunosuppressive agent, such as azathioprine.

Subsequently, the immunologist commenced John on azathioprine. One week after commencing this agent, John developed chills, muscle aches, lethargy and back pain. There were elevations of liver enzymes (ALP 188 U/L, reference <110 U/L; GGT 575 U/L, reference <60 U/L; and ALT 620 U/L, reference <55 U/L). The immunologist ceased azathioprine and advised John to avoid azathioprine in the future.

When John next saw the dermatologist, he considered itraconazole for the malassezia, but because of potential toxicity, he prescribed miconazole cream instead.

Despite the previous advice, Dr Roberts was still prescribing potent steroids for the face six years following the dermatologist's initial caution. There were never prescriptions for less potent steroids; Dr Roberts continued to prescribe oral steroids.

John consulted Dr Roberts on 74 occasions over 10 years. The medical record revealed almost continuous prescriptions for ocular steroids, and potent local steroids for the face and elsewhere. Dr Roberts recorded few other details about the conditions he was treating. He mentioned a facial rash on one occasion, and atopic dermatitis on the face and chest and dusty working conditions on another occasion. He noted previous immunotherapy and the need for moisturisers and emollients. When John was 32 Dr Roberts diagnosed allergic keratitis and prescribed steroid eye drops for three months.

At age 35, in mid summer, John presented with an itchy rash to a different general practitioner. The rash was worse in hot weather. There was an erythematous maculopapular eruption on the face, neck and upper chest. This second general practitioner noted that John had seen a dermatologist at some time in the past, and was commenced on a cortisone cream (details of potency of steroid and location of use were not recorded). There was no correspondence between this general practitioner and the dermatologist.

At age 36, John again consulted this second general practitioner, complaining of itchy red eyes, for which he had been using unspecified steroid and ciprofloxacin drops, utilising previous prescriptions from his usual doctor. He was prescribed olopatadine eye drops. Olopatadine is an H1 antagonist used for the treatment of seasonal allergic conjunctivitis. This practitioner suggested that John should see an ophthalmologist. John declined.

He returned four days later requesting prednisolone eye drops and told the practitioner that this usually worked better for him than the recently prescribed olopatadine. The doctor took a detailed history, including the fact that his usual general practitioner used a slit lamp, and had ruled out increased intraocular pressure. However, there was nothing in the general practice notes to suggest that intraocular pressure had been measured. John was counselled about the dangers of steroids, and given dexamethasone eye drops to be used for no more than four days.

John returned to the second doctor three months later, complaining of itchy eyes and nose as well as sneezing. He stated that the olopatadine had been ineffective, and that dexamethasone drops had been the only preparation able to relieve his symptoms. He requested and was prescribed dexamethasone eye drops, as well as 15 g of methylprednisolone aceponate ointment.

John repeated that he did not wish to see an ophthalmologist as his usual general practitioner checked his eyes. It was obvious that John had two different primary care medical providers, whose approaches to care were different from each other. There was no evidence that the second provider advised the first one of his reluctance to prescribe ophthalmic steroids.

The second general practitioner noted that John was quite forceful in his demands for ocular steroids. Against his better judgment this general practitioner acceded to John's request. It is possible that if the second general practitioner had communicated with the dermatologist, John would have avoided some of his long-term complications of excessive and inappropriate steroid use.

Eight months later John returned once more to his second doctor, and complained that he perceived the presence of a foreign body in his eye. The doctor, who was unable to detect a foreign body, wrote a referral to an ophthalmologist, for advice about chronic conjunctivitis.

This second general practitioner counselled John about the undesirability of his continuing in his current dusty employment. John stated that he did not wish to change his job, as he was self-employed and was running his own business.

Three weeks later the ophthalmologist diagnosed glaucoma secondary to long-term use of steroid eye drops. He also noted the use of the potent steroid creams, betamethasone, mometasone furoate and methylprednisolone aceponate. He commenced John on latanoprost and brimonidine eye drops and referred him to a consultant ophthalmologist specialising in glaucoma management.

The glaucoma specialist noted the history and medications, and commented that the therapy prescribed by the previous ophthalmologist had reduced the ocular pressures (right eye from 49 mmHg to 12 mmHg, left eye from 45 mmHg to 10 mmHg, reference 12–22 mmHg). She also commented that John had had tunnel vision for the previous five months, due to glaucoma. The diagnosis was advanced bilateral steroid response glaucoma.

The second ophthalmologist referred John to a second dermatologist, who managed to achieve control of his allergic diathesis. To complicate matters, the ophthalmologist discovered malassezia affecting both eyes. This was treated with locally applied itraconazole.

During the following two years John attended 12 ophthalmologist appointments and underwent four eye operations to control his ocular pressures and preserve his vision. His ocular pressure became satisfactory in the left eye, as did his vision. In the right eye his pressure remained around 22 mmHg, with his best vision being 6/9. At the time of writing, further surgery to the right eye was planned.

John is currently unable to work and is in receipt of a disability pension.

Legal Issues

In 2013 John commenced legal action for inappropriate medical care and loss of his employment. One of the reasons for his displeasure was that, if he had understood the potential gravity of his situation at an earlier time, he would have been able to retrain for different employment. His current medical condition significantly limited his options. The case is ongoing.

Discussion

During the timeframe of these events the pharmacist had supplied John with steroid eye drops on no fewer than 99 occasions, almost all on receipt of prescriptions from his original general practitioner, with a small number coming from the second general practitioner and the others involved in his care. There were 70 prescriptions for potent steroid creams and a total of 150 5 mg prednisolone tablets.

Corticosteroids applied to the skin may cause skin atrophy and fragility, and may be absorbed to a greater or lesser degree, depending on the site of application. Long-term application of potent steroid creams or ointments to the face, flexures, scrotum and intertriginous areas is contraindicated, as absorption may readily occur, leading to local and systemic side effects. A relatively safe steroid for facial application is hydrocortisone.

Steroids applied to the conjunctiva are likely to cause increased intraocular pressure, and must be used sparingly and with great care. Dr Roberts did not understand that.

Another issue that needed to be explored was the wisdom or otherwise of John continuing in his usual employment with his long-term skin condition. It should have been obvious to Dr Roberts and to the dermatologist that John's skin was incompatible with the demands of his employment, and vigorous efforts should have been made to counsel John about the need for retraining. Even though this would have involved a major reconstruction of John's working life, it would have seemed necessary for his health. There is no evidence that such a need was ever discussed, other than by the second general practitioner, whom John saw on several occasions.

Clinical Principles

It is well understood that potent steroids are contraindicated for long-term facial use. Dr Roberts must have been taught this. If he was unsure of the rationale for this advice, it would have been a simple matter to discover why it was so. Information was available online, and in textbooks, and from experienced general practice and specialist colleagues.

Long-term steroid use is contraindicated in or around the eyes, flexor regions and genitalia.

The first dermatologist did not discover that John had used conjunctival steroids, either because he did not ask the right questions about medications, or because John did not reveal this when asked. Careful history taking would likely have permitted earlier ophthalmologic consultation and intervention to reduce intraocular pressure.

There is no documentary evidence that Dr Roberts or the dermatologist counselled John to seek alternative employment. John's working environment was almost certainly detrimental to his welfare.

SAGGING LIP

History

When Elizabeth Paskin, aged 46, woke one morning in 2000, her husband noticed that the right side of her lips had sagged. She visited her local general practitioner, Dr Ana Surubian at 09:30 h, by which time the paresis had almost resolved and there was no other objective neurological finding. Elizabeth was a smoker with a family history of cerebrovascular disease.

Elizabeth had a history of long-standing muscle spasms at the right shoulder and neck. She attributed this to frequent tilting of her head to the right to reach the phone whilst constantly using a computer at work. Dr Surubian suggested physiotherapy to manage the spasms, and advised paracetamol to relieve the temporary symptoms.

Dr Surubian's record of the 09:30 h consultation referred to very minimal lip sagging on the right side, without any numbness at that time. She recorded that Elizabeth had said the skin at the right of her lips had felt swollen earlier, and that this sensation had reduced, but was still present at the time of the consultation. Dr Surubian noted that cranial nerve function was normal (which was inconsistent with her findings of paraesthesia and weakness). Dr Surubian considered that Elizabeth's symptoms might have been related to the right-sided muscular spasms of the neck and shoulder girdle. She syringed Elizabeth's ear, as it had a collection of cerumen.

Elizabeth returned home. When her children arrived home from school seven hours later, she was unable to get out of bed because she had suffered a dense left-sided hemiparesis. Elizabeth spent two months in hospital and further time in outpatient rehabilitation. Elizabeth is still unable to perform housework, to care for her children, or to resume work.

The left-sided paresis was due to right cerebral hemispheric ischaemia following embolisation of thrombus from the right internal carotid artery to the right middle cerebral artery.

Legal Issues

Elizabeth complained about the standard of care offered by Dr Surubian. The expert witness general practitioner for the plaintiff opined that Dr Surubian's assessment was inadequate, and that this denied Elizabeth the opportunity to receive treatment in hospital which may have prevented her debilitating stroke.

The expert witness general practitioner for the defence did not attach any significance to her history of neurological symptoms and said that further investigation was not warranted. The other defence witness, a distinguished neurologist at a capital city teaching hospital, stated that urgent referral was unnecessary, and that some consultant neurologists would fail to recognise the significance of Elizabeth's symptoms and signs. He opined that if all patients with a neck disorder were referred for neurological assessment they would be accused of overservicing.

The matter settled at mediation.

Discussion

This apparently uncomplicated clinical problem raises two important issues. In recent years there has been a reduction of time available at medical schools to teach anatomy generally, and neuroanatomy in particular. Time available to teach newer subjects in the curriculum has been gained at the expense of time available to teach anatomy. This reduction in the teaching of anatomy has probably been an impediment to recent graduates' understanding of the mechanisms of problems such as Elizabeth's.

Dr Surubian conflated shoulder and neck spasms with lip paraesthesia and paresis, because she did not understand the neuroanatomy of the region.

The fifth cranial nerve supplies sensation to the superficial and deep parts of the face, and is a motor nerve to the muscles of mastication. The seventh cranial nerve, a mixed sensory and motor nerve, supplies the superficial muscles of the face and neck. The muscles of the shoulder are supplied by the anterior primary rami of the fifth and sixth cervical nerves and the first dorsal nerve via branches of the cervical plexus.

Since the nerve supply to the shoulder has no relationship to the nerve supply of the lips, Elizabeth's neck and lip symptoms could not have a common cause. The symptoms and signs which were present at 09:30 h were most likely due to irritation of the right fifth and seventh cranial nerves. Elizabeth required urgent management at the local accident and emergency department. She did not require paracetamol and elective physiotherapy.

What is the explanation for right facial paraesthesia and weakness in the morning, and left hemiparesis later in the day? The internal carotid artery within the cranium is adjacent to the fifth and seventh cranial nerves as they emerge from the brain. Irritation of these nerves is likely to have occurred as a result of inflammation around the right internal carotid artery, causing altered sensation and drooping of the lips on the right side; subsequent occlusion of the right middle cerebral artery caused the left hemiparesis. It is possible, but less likely, that right facial paraesthesia and weakness were related to a vascular disturbance to the left side of the brain.

The second important issue is the responsibility of expert witnesses to provide honest and unbiased reports to assist the court. This involves having regard to all of the evidence, including the objective evidence of examinations made by practitioners at the time of the relevant events. In this case the court had to decide the merits of Elizabeth's claim.

The plaintiff's expert witness general practitioner analysed the problem based on the documentation provided to him. His opinion, taking account of the evidence, was that Elizabeth should have been referred immediately to the hospital emergency department. It was inappropriate to send Elizabeth home for elective physiotherapy.

The expert witness general practitioner engaged by the defence played down the history of altered sensation of the lip, ignored the asymmetry of the lips observed by the general practitioner, and said he did not consider immediate investigation in hospital was indicated.

The expert witness neurologist engaged by the defence concentrated on the possible management of Elizabeth if she had been referred to an emergency department, and the possible impediments to proper management. He did not suggest that urgent referral was necessary, and commented that some neurologists would fail to recognise the significance of the symptoms and signs, and would not arrange early investigations. If true, that would indicate a poor understanding of neuroanatomy amongst some physicians trained as consultant neurologists. This is unlikely to be the case.

Clinical Principles

It is difficult to understand why Dr Surubian suggested that Elizabeth take paracetamol for her condition, as there seemed no rational explanation for this.

As long as medical schools do not give students an adequate grounding in anatomy, patients such as Elizabeth will risk poor management.

Two of the expert witnesses, engaged to assist the court, did not address the urgent management issue and one did not have proper regard to the totality of the medical history taken at the time of treatment. These witnesses failed to fulfil their obligation to provide complete and unbiased assessments for the benefit of the court. Their opinions seemed to favour the objectives of the legal firm who appointed them to analyse the issues; their opinions were arguably not unbiased.

TONGUE CANCER

History

In 2014 at the age 56, Deepak Sharma gradually developed a right-sided earache. Deepak was a keen scuba diver and thought it might be due to an ear infection from being frequently in the water. He tried Aquaear ear drops, but it did not help. After a few weeks, he decided to consult his general practitioner.

Deepak saw his general practitioner, Dr Arnav Vengsarkar, on 2 November 2014. Dr Vengsarkar could not see any abnormality. He referred Deepak to ear, nose and throat (ENT) surgeon, Dr Albert Cunningham.

Deepak first consulted Dr Cunningham on 1 December 2014. Dr Cunningham obtained a history of right earache aggravated by chewing. He also obtained a history of daily alcohol consumption with occasional heavy bouts of drinking. He examined Deepak's oropharynx and larynx with the use of a headlamp as well as a flexible laryngoscope. He palpated Deepak's neck, but did not, according to Deepak, palpate his tongue or any other part of his mouth. Dr Cunningham diagnosed a low-grade middle ear infection for which he prescribed antibiotics.

The right-sided earache persisted. It was not severe, but troublesome enough for Deepak to see his general practitioner on a few occasions for which he was prescribed further courses of antibiotics. He saw a dentist, who could find no dental cause for the pain. There were no identifiable problems with Deepak's temporomandibular joint.

After about one year of putting up with the symptoms, Deepak asked his general practitioner to refer him back to Dr Cunningham for review. By the time of the referral on 8 November 2015, Deepak had developed a sore throat over the preceding few months and a feeling that he had ulcers on the back of his tongue.

On 5 December 2015, Deepak again saw Dr Cunningham. Dr Cunningham obtained a history of right-sided otalgia from 2014, which was aggravated by chewing and swallowing, together with a sore throat and a feeling that he had ulcers on the back of his tongue. Dr Cunningham examined Deepak's oropharynx and larynx and palpated Deepak's neck. He used a flexible laryngoscope, but did not palpate the base of Deepak's tongue. He could find no abnormality. Thinking that he may be missing something occult, Dr Cunningham ordered a CT scan of the soft tissues of the neck.

The CT scan was performed the next day and reported as showing mild tonsillar enlargement, sinusitis, but no other abnormality. Deepak returned to see Dr Cunningham on 10 December 2015. Dr Cunningham found no abnormality and reported to Deepak that the CT scan was normal. He advised Deepak and Dr Vengsarkar that there was nothing further he could do and advised Deepak to see a dentist.

Over the next six months, Deepak had worsening right-sided ear pain, and a sore throat. He consulted a number of dentists, but no cause was found.

On 10 May 2016, Deepak was again referred back to Dr Cunningham by Dr Vengsarkar. He performed the same examination and prescribed Panadeine Forte and a nonsteroidal antiinflammatory drug.

By July 2016, Deepak had lost weight and had developed pain in the right side of his jaw with numbness radiating to the right side of his face. Dr Vengsarkar referred Deepak to a neurologist, Dr Colin Smith.

Deepak consulted Dr Smith on 14 August 2016. He obtained a history of progressively worsening right earache, sore throat, difficulty chewing and swallowing, an altered taste in the mouth, weight loss and slurred speech. On examination, Deepak had weakness and fasciculations of the tongue. Dr Smith investigated a neurogenic cause for the symptoms, including electromyography and an MRI scan of the brain. These were negative. He then ordered a CT scan of the soft tissues of the neck, which demonstrated a heterogeneous abnormality of the base of the tongue. The radiologist recommended an MRI scan of the soft tissues of the neck and the base of the tongue.

The MRI scan suggested there was a malignancy of the base of the tongue. Deepak was referred to an oral and maxillofacial surgeon, Dr George Franklin. He ordered a PET scan, which demonstrated a base of tongue mass consistent with a high-grade cancer with extension to the floor of the mouth and local lymph nodes.

On 16 November 2016, Dr Franklin performed a tongue biopsy, which revealed an adenoid cystic carcinoma of the tongue. The next day, Deepak underwent a total glossectomy and lymph node dissection.

After recovering from the operation, he had difficulty communicating and eating, and was embarrassed by the loss of his tongue.

Two years later, Deepak was diagnosed with locoregional recurrence as well as pulmonary metastases. His life expectancy is dramatically reduced.

LEGAL ISSUES

In 2018, Deepak gave instructions to commence proceedings against Dr Cunningham for failing promptly to diagnose his base of tongue cancer. Based upon independent expert ENT opinion, Deepak alleged that the base of tongue cancer was present and diagnosable on 1 December 2015 and at all times he saw Dr Cunningham. He alleged that the failure to palpate the base of his tongue was negligent. If the base of the tongue had been palpated, then an abnormality would have been detected, which would have led to appropriate imaging, earlier diagnosis and different treatment. He also alleged that a generalised or nonspecific CT scan of the soft tissues of the neck was an inappropriate investigation to confirm or exclude a base of tongue cancer.

Dr Cunningham obtained expert ENT evidence contrary to that advanced by Deepak. The expert considered that Dr Cunningham's examination was reasonable and that the CT scan of the soft tissues of the neck was an appropriate screening examination. The expert was provided with assumptions on which he based his opinion. Those assumptions were that, although Dr Cunningham could not remember any of the consultations, in keeping with his usual practice, he would have palpated the base of Deepak's tongue at each consultation. This is because he was likely to have considered a base of tongue cancer as a differential diagnosis in light of Deepak's presenting symptoms. Thus, there was a factual contest between Deepak's recollection of there being no tongue palpation and Dr Cunningham's evidence of his usual practice of performing such an examination.

The ENT expert evidence was that Deepak would have avoided a total glossectomy with earlier diagnosis. The base of tongue cancer would have been able to be resected without removing the whole of his tongue. There would also have been no metastases.

There was a dispute between oncologists relied on by both parties as to whether earlier diagnosis would have made a difference to outcome.

The oncologists agreed that there had been upgrading of a part of the adenoid cystic carcinoma over time. One oncologist thought that it occurred late so that earlier diagnosis would have resulted in treatment of a less aggressive cancer. The alternative view was that Deepak became symptomatic in December 2015 because there had already been transformation to a poorly differentiated carcinoma, which meant Deepak's prognosis was poor even if the cancer had been diagnosed earlier. Dr Cunningham's expert was aware of Deepak's history of alcohol consumption and so suggested that Dr Cunningham's failure to diagnose made no difference to Deepak's outcome.

The case settled at mediation.

Discussion

Dr Cunningham accepted that he ought to have considered a base of tongue cancer among his differential diagnoses because of the chronic and progressive nature of Deepak's symptoms, especially the onset of a sore throat and a feeling of having ulcers on the back of the tongue. The contest was in relation to the nature of the examinations performed by Dr Cunningham and the adequacy of a nonspecific CT scan of the soft tissues of the neck in excluding a base of tongue cancer.

There are often contests in medicolegal proceedings about what was said during a consultation or what examination was performed. Understandably, an individual patient is much more likely to remember the details of a consultation than a medical practitioner, who may see many patients per day. With the effluxion of time, the likelihood of a doctor remembering a particular consultation becomes remote. In the circumstances, the quality of medical record keeping is very important in determining what actually happened. Medical practitioners often do not help their cause by having deficient records.

Dr Cunningham made no note about palpating the base of Deepak's tongue. While he visually inspected the area with the flexible laryngoscope, an occult lump may not be visualised unless there was also a surface abnormality. Deepak's tumour was slow growing until there was dedifferentiation. Palpation may have given more information than direct visualisation. Defendant medical practitioners often argue (or at least their lawyers argue) that they record only positive examination findings rather than negative findings in their notes. Such an argument was unavailable to Dr Cunningham because his notes recorded the absence of abnormalities with some of the other examinations he performed such as palpation of the neck. Often, negative findings are as important as positive findings in coming to a diagnosis so the practice of selective recording is potentially dangerous.

If there is no recollection of a consultation and the clinical records do not help refresh the recollection, it is sometimes open for a medical practitioner to rely on his or her usual practice. The assumption is that, if a person generally does something often, then it is likely that that step would have been taken in the circumstances of an individual case. It is not always possible to refute an assertion based upon usual practice. It was unclear how a trial judge would have determined the dispute between Deepak's actual recollection and Dr Cunningham's reliance on his usual practice of palpating the base of the tongue. In any event, there was no guarantee that palpation would have led to detection of an abnormality.

Accordingly, the case boiled down to the need to perform more specific imaging such as a thin slice CT scan through the base of the tongue, an MRI scan or a positron emission tomogram (PET) scan. Dr Cunningham's expert asserted that a nonspecific CT scan of the soft tissues was reasonable. Deepak's ENT expert agreed it was a reasonable screening tool, but if negative could not be relied on as excluding occult cancer at the base of the tongue. As his peers supported his conduct, Dr Cunningham may well have been found to have acted in accordance with proper peer professional practice by only ordering a general CT scan.

Clinical Principles

In many of the cases in which we have been involved, after considering serious pathology as a differential diagnosis, a doctor has ordered an investigation to confirm or exclude that pathology. Often, however, the investigation ordered is a screening test such as a CT scan without contrast of the brain for intracranial pathology or, as here, a nonspecific CT scan of the soft tissues of the neck for a possible base of tongue lesion. Dr Cunningham appeared to believe that a general CT scan would exclude a base of tongue cancer. The premise appears to have been that, if there were a cancer, then it would be large enough to be apparent on such a scan. The argument only needs to be stated to be rejected as fallacious. If a doctor is serious about excluding certain pathology, then it is sometimes necessary to go beyond a screening test.

While there is always a balance between cost and benefit, it is unlikely serious pathology can always be excluded by a screening test. A screening test is useful if it demonstrates an abnormality. But the same weight cannot be attached to a negative result. For many cancers, the prognosis is better with early diagnosis and treatment. That opportunity should not be missed by failing to understand how to interpret screening tests.

CHILDHOOD CANCER

History

At the age of 13, Mary Kilpatrick, was diagnosed with an undifferentiated soft tissue sarcoma at the C7 vertebral level. She commenced chemoradiation treatment at a specialist hospital for children under the care of paediatric oncologist, Professor Michael Harrington.

The cancer was diagnosed after a debulking operation by an experienced neurosurgeon in February 1989. He performed a right-sided C6-7 laminectomy and found the tumour surrounding the C7 nerve roots and extending proximally to just inside the dura mater. It extended laterally to the intervertebral canal. The neurosurgeon removed the extradural tumour and part of the tumour that had penetrated the dura mater. The surgical specimens were sent to the pathology department where the tumour was diagnosed as a primitive neuroectodermal tumour, also known as an extraosseous Ewing's sarcoma.

Professor Harrington was responsible for prescribing the chemotherapeutic agents, including their dose, route of administration and timing in relation to the radiotherapy Mary also received.

Mary received 46 Gy of radiation (XRT) to C2–T2 in 26 fractions over 37 days. She received a boost of 2 Gy in April, followed by intravenous systemic chemotherapy in the form of vincristine, cyclophosphamide and actinomycin-D. She also received intrathecal treatment known as triple intrathecal chemotherapy (TIT) where the chemotherapeutic drugs were injected into the cerebrospinal fluid around her spinal cord. The TIT comprised methotrexate, cytosine arabinoside and hydrocortisone. TIT was prescribed because the sarcoma had penetrated the dura mater surrounding the spinal cord.

Mary's treatment was very aggressive. The chemotherapeutic agents administered were toxic. In the context of a life-threatening malignancy, this was understandable.

The treatment regimen was based on old guidelines published by the Intergroup Rhabdomyosarcoma Study Group (IRSG), which was the world's peak research group in relation to soft tissue sarcomas, at the time. The IRSG regularly published its research findings and recommendations for treatment in peer-reviewed journals. It had amended its guidelines for the treatment of soft tissue sarcomas in 1987 (protocol IRS-3) by abandoning TIT because of the risk of transverse myelitis.

At the time he prescribed the course of treatment for Mary, Professor Harrington was unaware of the change to the IRS-3 protocol. One of the paediatric oncologists from the hospital, however, had attended a meeting run by IRSG where the risks of TIT had been discussed. He had not communicated the new recommendations to Professor Harrington.

The XRT was administered in weeks one to three and weeks five to six. Mary received TIT in weeks two, three, five and thirteen. Three courses of TIT were delivered during the course of XRT. One course of intrathecal methotrexate (on its own) was delivered during XRT. Systemic chemotherapy with actinomycin-D was administered in week 20. The combination of some chemotherapy agents potentiates the effect of the radiation.

By week 21 of treatment, Mary developed a cervical myelopathy in the form of transverse myelitis. The inflammation of the spinal cord was directly related to the TIT, particularly its concurrent administration with XRT.

Although treatment ceased as soon as the diagnosis was made, Mary was left a permanent quadriplegic. She was, however, cured of her sarcoma.

Legal Issues

Mary commenced proceedings in the Supreme Court in 1993. Her case went to trial in 2005. She sued Professor Harrington and the local area health service. The principal allegation was that she should not have been prescribed TIT at the doses she received, on the basis that the scientific literature relevant to the treatment of her tumour had indicated that TIT should no longer be used because of a significant risk of myelitis associated with its use.

A number of paediatric oncologists and radiation oncologists provided opinions. It was accepted that it was reasonable to consider TIT given the location of the tumour and its invasion into the dura mater. Mary's case was that proper consideration should have led to the exclusion of TIT from her treatment regimen because of the changes to the IRS-3 protocol. Mary also alleged that, even if it were reasonable to prescribe TIT, the doses given were excessive given she received concurrent XRT at the maximum dose possible. All these issues were disputed by the defendants.

At first instance, the judge found for Mary against the local area health service, but not against Professor Harrington. The local area health service appealed and Mary cross-appealed against Professor Harrington. In 2006, the Court of Appeal allowed Mary's appeal and disallowed the local area health service's appeal. The upshot was that judgment was entered against both the local area health service and Professor Harrington.

Discussion

The case was principally about a failure to fulfil a professional's continuing obligation to keep himself or herself informed about the management of the conditions he or she treats. Professor Harrington neither kept himself up-to-date with the current protocols for the treatment of soft tissue sarcomas of the type Mary suffered nor the risks associated with their treatment. This meant that Mary was administered outmoded and toxic TIT for her sarcoma and developed transverse myelitis and quadriplegia as a result.

The TIT should not have been given or alternatively should not have been given at the dose and frequency Mary received. Eighteen months prior to her diagnosis, the premier international research group into sarcomas, the IRSG, had significantly reduced its recommended doses for TIT and XRT because of the risk of life-threatening neurotoxicity. Professor Harrington was not aware of this change. One of his colleagues had attended a conference, but had not passed on this information to Professor Harrington. It is likely that Mary would have been cured of her cancer and survived without any neurological damage if she had not received TIT.

Given the serious and potentially lethal risks that were associated with treatment of childhood cancers, Professor Harrington and the local area health service's management required a degree of diligence that, as far as possible, guaranteed the prescription of treatment in accordance with the most current and considered guidelines available in the world. This did not happen.

Medical practitioners must keep themselves abreast of the scientific literature relevant to the conditions they diagnose and treat. It also highlights the fact that, when dealing with particularly harmful conditions or treatment, the duty requires an additional diligence to be proactive in the management of the condition.

Clinical Principles

Although Mary suffered from a rare tumour, this did not mean that Professor Harrington and the local area health service could be excused for not getting the treatment regimen right. The site of the cancer was important not only in relation to survival but also in relation to the type of therapy that had to be instituted. The IRSG advised TIT only for sarcomas involving the cranial meninges. It was not recommended for paraspinal sarcomas even if there was meningeal extension as in Mary's case. While the treatment of childhood malignancies is an emotional and difficult task, there was nonetheless a need to be careful in the selection of the treatment regimen and to be fully informed of any changes to protocols for treatment.

NECK PAIN

History

Barry Grant worked as a storeman for a major retail company. In October 2009, at the age of 31, Barry's left foot was run over by a forklift at work, causing a laceration but no fracture. His general practitioner cleaned, dressed and bandaged the wound, and prescribed antibiotics.

Two weeks later Barry consulted his general practitioner complaining of neck and back pain of one week's duration. On examination, there was tenderness over the cervical spine from C3 to C7. The doctor ordered a plain x-ray of the cervical spine, which revealed no abnormality. The neck and back pain persisted. As a result, his general practitioner referred Barry to the emergency department at the local hospital.

Barry had a somewhat checkered career. He had not worked consistently after leaving school and the jobs he found were varied. He had not developed any genuine skills to hold him in good stead should serious illness or injury arise. He also had a history over five to ten years of using heroin and amphetamine, and had reused and shared needles.

In the emergency department at the hospital, Barry was assessed by the triage nurse at 15:20 h, who recorded a one week history of pain between the shoulder blades and in the neck associated with a reduced range of motion in his neck and shoulder, without any headaches, nausea, vomiting or problems with mobility. The pain was aggravated by coughing and lying flat. Barry's pulse rate was 92/min with an oxygen saturation of 97% breathing room air. His temperature was 39.2°C. He had not taken any antiinflammatory drug prior to presentation. At 18:36 h, he was given two tablets of paracetamol with codeine. Barry's vital signs were monitored while he was in the emergency department. At one point, his pulse rate increased up to 130/min. His temperature had gone down by the time he was examined by a medical practitioner.

At 19:25 h, Barry was examined by a resident medical officer, Dr Amy Wong, who obtained a history of neck and back pain coming on one week after the left foot injury. There were no neurological symptoms. Barry also told her of his past use of illicit drugs and that he had a sore throat. On examination, Dr Wong found cervical spinal tenderness and a limited range of movement in the neck, particularly with flexion and extension. The range of movement was limited by pain. Oropharyngeal examination was normal.

Dr Wong's diagnosis was musculoskeletal pain; she advised Barry to take regular analgesia and to return to his general practitioner for follow-up. She suggested a CT scan or MRI scan of the spine if the pain did not resolve.

Barry followed Dr Wong's advice. He returned to his general practitioner the next week with persistent pain, and a sore throat. The pain was in the neck radiated to the thoracic spine, and was not relieved by regular paracetamol. The general practitioner found muscle tenderness on the left side of the neck with a decreased range of cervical movement. He diagnosed bilateral neck pain and left shoulder pain and ordered an ultrasound to test for possible tendonitis. The ultrasound was normal.

Barry's pain continued and increased in severity. Two weeks after the ultrasound he suddenly lost sensation and power in his legs, and was taken by ambulance to the emergency department at the local hospital. At presentation, he gave a history of four weeks' neck pain, which had increased in severity. He told staff that the pain was associated with sensory and motor deficits from the hips down. He had tingling in the feet and hands, reduced sensation in all limbs and had not passed urine since the acute deterioration that day. He could not stand. On examination, there was decreased sensation and reduced power in the upper limbs, no power in the lower limbs, and absent reflexes and sensation below the T4 level. He was febrile.

As part of a septic work-up, blood was taken for microscopy and culture. It grew methicillin-resistant staphylococcus aureus (MRSA). Barry was transferred to a tertiary hospital, where he had an MRI scan. The diagnosis was a spinal epidural abscess (SEA) spanning C5 to C7 with retropharyngeal space extension and associated C5/6 discitis and osteomyelitis. The spinal canal was narrowed by approximately 50%, causing cord compression and oedema.

Barry underwent emergency decompression surgery one month after his initial presentation. Despite antibiotic treatment and surgical drainage of the abscess, Barry remained a C5 level quadriparetic. He also developed a central neuropathic pain syndrome for which he was prescribed gabapentin.

Legal Issues

Barry commenced proceedings in negligence against the local area health service that conducted the emergency department at his local hospital, because of avoidable neurological deficit. There was a dispute as to whether the initial pyrexia recorded in the notes was part of Barry's records or part of another patient's records. An infectious diseases physician argued that there was no reason to think Barry's initial presentation was in any way due to an infective process. The defendant maintained that in the absence of evidence of pyrexia, there was no need to take Barry's temperature as part of routine observations of a patient presenting to an emergency department with neck pain. The infectious diseases physician did not dispute the likelihood of there being an elevated temperature if it had been measured, in light of what was known about the actual illness responsible for Barry's presentation.

The opinions of expert witnesses relied on by the plaintiff (an infectious diseases physician, an emergency medicine specialist and a neurosurgeon) agreed that there was a probable infectious process causing Barry cervical pain. Barry's temperature would more likely than not have been elevated, if it had been measured.

The matter settled at mediation.

Discussion

SEA may result from direct spread from local infection or, more often, via haematogenous seeding from a site of infection elsewhere in the body. In Barry's case, it was likely that the cut to his left foot at work was the portal of entry for the MRSA. As he was an intravenous drug user, he was particularly susceptible to infection, which meant that staff at the emergency department at his local hospital, including Dr Wong, should have been vigilant to exclude an infective cause for his presentation.

SEA is a neurosurgical emergency. It can only be diagnosed with confidence by an MRI scan. The only effective form of treatment is surgical drainage and antibiotic therapy. The aim of neurosurgery is to halt progression of the neurological deficits. If SEA is diagnosed and treated before major neurological problems develop, then prognosis is optimised and there may be minimal permanent disability.

In Barry's case, he sought attention early on in the course of his SEA, well before the final, rapid deterioration with spinal cord damage and obvious neurological deficits. While a benign cause for his neck pain was reasonably entertained at the outset, the diagnosis of a musculoskeletal problem became untenable with the persistence of neck pain past his two consultations with his general practitioner. It was appreciated in retrospect that the development of a sore throat was likely to be due to retropharyngeal extension of the abscess.

If the diagnosis had been suspected by Dr Wong based on neck pain and tenderness one week after an open foot history, Barry would have undergone an MRI one month earlier than was the case. He would have been diagnosed as suffering from a SEA, and would have undergone decompression surgery. He more likely than not would have avoided progression to quadriparesis.

Clinical Principles

Firstly, Barry's case demonstrates the importance of history taking. Barry reported a recent foot injury and intravenous drug use, and these were both red flags for an infective cause of his neck pain. Both of these red flags ought to have been recognised by the emergency department doctors.

The case highlights the importance of excluding an organic basis for a presentation involving pain before attributing it to a mechanical or musculoskeletal problem of no specificity.

It also serves as an example of how Occam's razor (among competing hypotheses, the one with the fewest assumptions should be selected) may be applied to medical diagnosis and problem-solving. It was simpler to explain Barry's neck pain, restricted movement and pyrexia by one cause rather than invoking multiple separate processes such as mechanical pain, an upper respiratory tract infection to account for the sore throat and an unrelated left foot injury two weeks prior to presentation.

SHOULDER PAIN

HISTORY

Shirley Finney was 35 years old when she presented to Dr Boris Sokolov, a general practitioner she had not seen previously. Shirley had a history of substance abuse that she stated had ceased 10 years prior to the events of 2004.

Shirley had systemic lupus erythematosus, which her longstanding general practitioner had managed well, with prednisone as required. Shirley's usual doctor declined to prescribe the increasing amounts of benzodiazepines that she requested, so she found a more compliant practitioner.

Shirley presented to Dr Sokolov in January 2004 complaining of headaches and pain to her right shoulder and right upper limb. The only notes recorded by Dr Sokolov at this consultation were that Shirley had stated that she suffered from lupus, and that prednisone 5 mg, diazepam 5 mg and alprazolam 2 mg had been prescribed.

Shirley visited Dr Sokolov three weeks later; he noted lupus, severe pain and that she was a former heroin addict. He provided prescriptions for tramadol 50 mg and diazepam 5 mg, and requested a full blood count. The white cell count was 14.0×10^9/L (reference $4.3–10.8 \times 10^9$/L), with 12.6×10^9/L neutrophils (reference $1.5–8.0 \times 10^9$/L).

Shirley revisited Dr Sokolov three days later with the same symptoms. In addition she reported that she found walking difficult because of ataxia, to the extent that she required two persons to support her. She had severe neck pain, slurred speech and intense abdominal pain. Dr Sokolov wrote prescriptions for oral tramadol 200 mg, diazepam 5 mg, amoxycillin 250 mg and morphine 30 mg × 5 (one box), for injection.

The following day Shirley arrived at a tertiary referral teaching hospital by ambulance. The records refer to her being unwell for the past week, a possible chest infection, left sided chest pain worse on inspiration, whitish sputum and left sided axillary pain.

The emergency department doctor noted that she was not tachypnoeic. Her temperature was 36.6°C. She had crepitations at the left lower zone with dullness to percussion. The chest x-ray demonstrated an opacity left lower zone. The presumptive diagnosis was pneumonia. Shirley was admitted and treated initially with cefuroxime and roxithromycin, later changed to intravenous clarithromycin and ampicillin. The white cell count on admission was 15.4×10^9/L with 13.0×10^9/L neutrophils.

The following day the hospital doctor wrote "patient unsteady on her feet. Having a lot of pain and aches". He did not examine Shirley. On the same day the occupational therapist referred to her unsteadiness and the need to use a walking stick. Several days later Shirley was discharged from the hospital.

The next week Shirley revisited Dr Sokolov, who noted generalised aches and pains, and a request for oral steroids. He prescribed prednisone, aspirin and diazepam. Two weeks later Shirley returned to Dr Sokolov with persistent neck and right arm pains, like electric shocks. He did not examine Shirley. Dr Sokolov diagnosed depression, and prescribed alprazolam, diazepam and amitriptyline.

One week later Shirley was found on the floor at home, unable to move. She told the ambulance officers her history of feeling dizzy and unsteady on her feet since her hospital admission one month earlier. She was readmitted to the same hospital. Her hepatitis C antibody positive status and other details (including pains and ataxia, and previous heroin use) were recorded.

The emergency department doctor performed a neurological examination. This was the first time a neurological assessment had been made since Shirley first reported neurological symptoms two weeks previously. In the event, the doctor did not consider that there was any significant neurological finding at the time. It was presumed that Shirley was ataxic following a seizure, although there was no evidence that she had had a seizure.

Shirley was reviewed by the medical registrar, who requested a septic work-up, but did not perform a neurological examination. Shirley reported reduced urinary output, blurred vision, inability to stand because of weakness to her legs and numbness of her legs. The white cell count was 14.7×10^9/L, and the C-reactive protein (CRP) was 45 mg/L (reference <5 mg/L). Shirley's symptoms worsened.

The consultant neurologist, who reviewed her the following day because of weakness in all limbs, concluded that she probably had an organic lesion at the C6 level. An MRI scan confirmed that there was an epidural phlegmon at C6/7 and osteophytes at C3/4, C4/5 and C5/6. Urgent neurosurgery was performed. Postoperatively, Shirley had permanent paralysis of the legs, with partial recovery of arm function over the following two years. She now lives in supported care.

Legal Issues

Shirley sought compensation for disability due to delayed diagnosis and treatment. The matter was settled at mediation.

Discussion

Although Shirley reported symptoms compatible with and suggestive of spinal abscess when she first consulted Dr Sokolov, the diagnosis was not made until three months later.

The first thing to note is Shirley's history of substance abuse that she claimed had ceased 10 years previously. An experienced practitioner should consider that a patient reporting previous substance abuse may be elastic with the truth. A patient with such a history, and neck pain, should be meticulously assessed for the possibility of a spinal abscess; this is the diagnosis until proven otherwise.

Dr Sokolov did not record an examination at any time, despite Shirley's varied and significant symptoms, and merely provided Shirley with what she requested. He prescribed benzodiazepines liberally, seemingly at Shirley's request. He even prescribed morphine for self-injection. Such behaviour indicated reckless indifference to Shirley's welfare.

Dr Sokolov displayed a totally inadequate standard of care in terms of assessment and management. All doctors who manage primary care patients, either in general practice or in the emergency department, should be able to perform and interpret a neurological examination. The reliance or over-reliance on sophisticated investigative modalities to make diagnoses is very much a retrograde step in patient management.

Dr Sokolov accepted Shirley's history of systemic lupus erythematosus without exploring the matter. She complained of intense abdominal pain and she was prescribed amoxicillin without any apparent rationale for that therapy. There seemed to be no consideration of the reason for her neck, shoulder and arm pain.

When Shirley was admitted to the hospital on the first occasion, even though her symptoms were recorded, no one performed a neurological examination. At the subsequent hospital admission, although there was evidence of infection, it was presumed that Shirley was ataxic following a seizure.

The emergency department doctor performed an incomplete neurological examination and diagnosed ataxia after a seizure. The medical registrar assessed her and suspected infection, but did not perform a neurological examination. Shirley's neurological symptoms worsened during the next 12 hours. By the time she was reviewed by a consultant neurologist, Shirley had permanent and disabling deficits.

Clinical Principles

The veracity of statements about current substance use by a patient with previous substance abuse must always be questioned. Such patients may attempt to confuse doctors so that they can obtain further supplies of what they want.

Doctors are obliged to consider carefully the circumstances of all clinical presentations. They must be alert to the risk of overlooking important symptoms and signs, particularly in patients who present recurrently.

Doctors must be careful not to neglect thoughtful and adequate physical examination and assessment of those who have a history of substance abuse or unusual manner of speech or physical appearance or state of personal hygiene or other factors.

As many wise clinicians have observed over the years, if one listens carefully to the patient, the diagnosis is often obvious, even before physical examination and investigations. Shirley's case demonstrates that this is not always appreciated.

UNEXPLAINED FEVER

History

One evening in 1997, Terry Gamell, aged 42, exercised as usual at the gymnasium. Over the previous three months or so he had felt somewhat lethargic, which was unusual for him. Several hours after his exercise, he developed a sudden severe pain in the left wrist, of such intensity that he took a total of six 500-mg-paracetamol combined with 30-mg-codeine tablets over a 10-hour period, with little relief. As well as this, he began to shiver uncontrollably, and huddled near to the gas heater to keep warm. During his shower the following morning, he felt giddy and almost collapsed. He believed that this collapse might have been related to the large amount of analgesia that he had consumed.

Instead of going to work, Terry presented to his long-term general practitioner, Dr Alan Lee, and described his symptoms. Dr Lee asked if he had injured his wrist. Terry said that he had exercised at the gymnasium the previous evening, as was his normal twice-weekly custom, and that nothing unusual had happened. He was convinced that the gymnasium attendance was not the reason for his discomfort.

Terry had been to the dentist twice recently, once three months previously, and again the day before his presentation with wrist pain. Dr Lee did not elicit this history.

Dr Lee detected tenderness at the base of the left thumb and over the distal end of the radius. He said that Terry had either strained his muscles at the gymnasium, or that he may have suffered an avulsion fracture.

Terry was still not confident that he had injured himself on the previous night, because the exercises were similar to his usual routine. Dr Lee explained that the rigors and feelings of hot and cold were being caused by a viral illness, even though he had not detected any evidence to suggest a viral illness, and had not recorded Terry's temperature.

An x-ray of the wrist revealed no bony abnormality. Dr Lee prescribed naproxen 1 g daily, advised Terry to use ice packs and suggested physiotherapy if he was not improving the next week. At his next consultation Terry told Dr Lee that he still had a fever, particularly at night. Dr Lee did not examine Terry.

Terry was increasingly uncomfortable the following day, and returned to the clinic where he saw a different general practitioner. Dr Lee's colleague limited his examination of Terry to the wrist only, and did not examine him more generally. He concluded that Terry was suffering with a tear of the intercarpal ligament, and provided a back-slab, additional pain relief, and advice to be reviewed three days later.

Ten days later, Terry attended the surgery once more, where he saw a third general practitioner. He reported that he was still taking the naproxen, was nauseated, and had suffered bilateral groin pain and fever for more than a week. The doctor detected slight tenderness over the lower abdomen, with normal renal areas, a blood pressure of 110/70 mmHg and ++ proteinuria. He arranged a urine culture and sensitivity, and advised Terry to increase his fluid intake, and to take a urinary alkalinisation powder four times per day. He concluded that Terry was suffering from a strain (site not specified) or a urinary tract infection. The urine culture was sterile.

A week later the wrist pain had lessened somewhat, but the other symptoms continued. Terry and his family went to the snowfields for two weeks for a previously arranged holiday. He was still feeling unwell with night sweats and fever and had not been enthusiastic about the proposed holiday. He hoped that the holiday and rest would aid in his recovery from the virus. While at the snow, the night sweats, weakness and lethargy persisted.

On his return from holidays he resumed work, however the wrist pain had returned, and he had developed left calf pain that caused him to limp.

Two weeks later he returned to the general practice clinic, complaining of left leg strain, muscle pains and continuing fever. The doctor on duty concluded that Terry did not have a thrombosis, and diagnosed tightness in the calf muscles, and pain in the thenar eminence. He prescribed paracetamol, and requested blood tests including those for Ross River virus.

On the way to the pathologist for his blood tests Terry collapsed because of a stroke affecting his right side.

The next entry by Dr Lee in Terry's medical record was written several weeks later. Terry had had acute bacterial endocarditis, with staphylococcus colonising his mitral valve, and a cerebral embolism, with right-sided weakness.

The records from the hospital referred to dental treatment three months prior to his stroke, and also on the day prior to his first visit to Dr Lee. Terry received four weeks of intravenous antibiotics, after which he was discharged from hospital. The diagnosis was bacterial endocarditis, with cerebral and radial artery embolism. Terry's convalescence in hospital was complicated by a further stroke, dense right hemiplegia, dysphasia and a pulmonary embolism.

Following discharge from the acute-care hospital, Terry was transferred to a rehabilitation hospital, where he remained for two months. A year after the initial episode Terry had persistent receptive and expressive dysphasia, although he was now able to read for short periods.

Memory and concentration were impaired, but less so than immediately following his stroke. Smell, taste and balance were disturbed, and he tended to fall to the right. There was persistent weakness in all muscles of the right arm and leg, and increased tendon reflexes.

Terry remained depressed, irritable and frustrated about his condition. His wife was unable to cope with the situation. Two years after the stroke they separated and Terry now lives alone. He occasionally sees his children. He is unable to work, and receives a disability pension. He still attends the same medical practice for ongoing care.

Legal Issues

Terry sought compensation for the consequences of delayed diagnosis and treatment of endocarditis. The case did not proceed to a court hearing and was settled at mediation.

Discussion

A basic principle of clinical practice is that if a patient presents with symptoms arising simultaneously from an array of body systems, these symptoms have a common genesis, unless it is obvious that this is not the case.

When Terry presented with rigors, wrist pain and fever, the correct approach was to eliminate potentially serious diagnoses. Differential diagnoses at first included infective endocarditis and other systemic illnesses. The history of recent dental work (and associated bacteraemia) increased the likelihood of endocarditis (in a patient with fever). Examination should have included general assessment including temperature, and focused attention to detect evidence of physical manifestations of endocarditis or other systemic illness. It was inappropriate to simply guess that Terry might have a viral infection.

There was no evidence that Dr Lee had taken a careful history. If he had asked Terry whether he had any recent illnesses or procedures, it is likely that the visits to the dentist would have been revealed. Then Terry would have been investigated and managed for endocarditis sooner than was the case, and stroke would have been avoided.

Dr Lee should have recorded Terry's temperature, and asked Terry to do the same at home before his next visit. This would have confirmed fever. A simple blood count would likely have suggested bacterial infection as the cause of fever. Blood cultures would have confirmed staphylococcal bacteraemia, and an echocardiogram would have demonstrated vegetation(s) on the mitral valve. Terry would have received appropriate intravenous antibiotics for six weeks, and the mitral valve would have been replaced during the period of antibiotic therapy. As it turned out, mitral valve replacement was contraindicated for at least several weeks because of the cerebral haemorrhagic risk associated with recent stroke.

It is unfortunate that none of the three doctors who saw Terry were sufficiently insightful as to look at the whole picture, rather than taking the approach of accepting the diagnosis of the first practitioner without further questioning.

The Australian, European and American colleges of general practice emphasise that the fundamental requirement of a general practitioner is to provide continuing, comprehensive, whole patient care.

Mistakes such as those in Terry's case may become more prevalent if practitioners consider the problems of patients in isolation, and do not invest sufficient time or effort to comply with their fundamental responsibility, to provide continuing comprehensive whole patient care. The development of large multidoctor clinics, where any one patient may be managed by an array of doctors with not one doctor taking overall management responsibility, is a recipe for error.

This is not to say that diagnostic errors may always be avoided if a single practitioner is responsible for care. Once a practitioner makes an incorrect diagnosis based on some clinical features, it is not uncommon for the same incorrect diagnosis to be made when a patient presents again with the same clinical features.

Was Terry's endocarditis acute or subacute at the time of presentation to Dr Lee? Terry had felt somewhat lethargic for some weeks prior to his first consultation with Dr Lee when he had wrist pain (this suggested subacute endocarditis). There was probably staphylococcal bacteraemia (more commonly associated with acute endocarditis) associated with mitral valve infection during the several months before onset of wrist pain. Pain at the wrist was due to arterial embolisation of infected material from the heart. Although there were features of both subacute and acute endocarditis, endocarditis of some sort should always have been on the list of differential diagnoses to explain Terry's symptoms.

Clinical Principles

The diagnosis of bacterial endocarditis is often delayed because initial symptoms are not considered to be due to a serious systemic illness such as endocarditis. It is always important to consider endocarditis in a patient with systemic symptoms including rigors or fever, in the context of previous dental, urogynaecological or gastrointestinal instrumentation. Endocarditis is often related to dental treatment involving the gums.

A comprehensive history, particularly in the presence of rigors, would have been likely to disclose the recent dental treatment, and led to early diagnosis and treatment.

The fundamental responsibility of a general practitioner is to provide continuing comprehensive whole patient care.

PERSISTENTLY UNWELL

HISTORY

Dawn Norville was aged 63 years in April 2013 when she became unwell with lethargy, fever and night sweats. For several years before this she had been under the care of Dr Osman Subahdar, cardiologist, following mechanical aortic valve replacement. In addition to anticoagulation with warfarin, her only other regular medication was amlodipine for hypertension. Dawn consulted her general practitioner a number of times and was prescribed several courses of oral antibiotics. Her CRP had been elevated before antibiotic therapy, but had fallen thereafter. She remained unwell. On 24 May 2013, she presented to hospital.

At the hospital, Dr Arjun Anand, emergency medicine specialist, noted that Dawn had been unwell for 6–8 weeks, initially with cough and dyspnoea, for which she had received antibiotics for a possible chest infection. She had increasing fatigue and reduced effort tolerance. Dr Anand wrote in Dawn's clinical notes that multiple courses of antibiotics may cloud the presentation of endocarditis, and that endocarditis should be considered to explain her illness. Blood was drawn for culture and other tests. The initial neutrophil count was 9.0×10^9/L (reference $2.0–7.0 \times 10^9$/L), with a leucocytosis (11.7×10^9/L, reference $4.0–10.0 \times 10^9$/L). The first CRP in hospital was not elevated (2.0 mg/L, reference <5.1 mg/L).

These results were discussed with Dr Subahdar, whose opinion was that endocarditis was unlikely in the absence of elevation of CRP. Dr Subahdar declined to have Dawn admitted under his care, and she was admitted to hospital somewhat surprisingly under the care of a gastroenterologist. Blood cultures were sterile. There was progressive neutrophil leucocytosis (see table below) and elevation of CRP (abnormal values in bold).

DATE	TIME	WHITE CELLS REFERENCE $4.0–10.0 \times 10^9$/L	NEUTROPHILS REFERENCE $2.0–7.0 \times 10^9$/L	CRP REFERENCE <5.1 mg/L
25 May	06:45	**11.7**	**9.0**	2.0
26 May	06:30	**13.2**	**10.8**	
27 May	05:15	**18.1**	**16.0**	4.5
27 May	09:10	**14.9**	**13.6**	**6.7**

Continued

DATE	TIME	WHITE CELLS REFERENCE 4.0–10.0 × 10^9/L	NEUTROPHILS REFERENCE 2.0–7.0 × 10^9/L	CRP REFERENCE <5.1 mg/L
27 May	15:29	**13.3**	**10.3**	
27 May	17:45	**15.8**	**14.3**	
28 May	00:33	**18.5**	**16.5**	
28 May	06:10	**16.0**	**14.0**	**48.1**
28 May	15:04	**16.2**	**13.5**	
28 May	17.29	**12.5**	**10.4**	
29 May	05:30	**15.2**	**13.3**	**146.0**
30 May	05:30	**11.8**	**9.0**	
31 May	05:45	8.0	6.4	
31 May	16:38	8.6	7.0	
01 June	05:30	**10.8**	**8.8**	
02 June	06:15	**11.3**	**9.8**	

During the morning of 26 May 2013 Dawn experienced double vision. When she was examined by the medical staff, they detected no neurological deficit, and wrote in the progress notes that endocarditis had been considered on admission, but that the diagnosis had been excluded because the CRP was not elevated. Nevertheless, a CT brain scan was appropriately requested. This showed an area of hypodensity in the right cerebellum, due to ischaemia.

The following morning Dawn was confused and on neurological examination there was now evidence of cerebellar dysfunction and intermittent diplopia. In the context of possible infective endocarditis, an echocardiogram was appropriately requested.

Dawn was reviewed by Dr Subahdar early on the afternoon of 27 May 2013. Although the CRP at 09:10 h that morning was now above the upper limit of normal, Dr Subahdar maintained that endocarditis was not likely because the CRP was normal and stable. The CRP was in fact neither normal nor stable. Despite Dr Subahdar's opinion, Dawn was transferred to a referral centre where neurosurgical and cardiac surgery were available.

A repeat CT brain scan showed multiple cerebellar hypodensities and evidence of raised intracranial pressure. The diagnosis now was right cerebellar infarction due to embolism from the aortic valve with or without haemorrhagic transformation. Dawn received broad spectrum intravenous antibiotics (vancomycin and gentamicin), and proceeded to posterior fossa evacuation and placement of a ventriculoperitoneal shunt. No vegetation was seen on a transoesophageal echocardiogram. Dawn did not improve clinically, and required a percutaneous tracheostomy. She died on 2 June 2013.

Legal Issues

Dawn's family sought compensation for the consequences of delayed diagnosis and treatment of endocarditis. They claimed damages for the loss of domestic services and for nervous shock.

A microbiologist expert witness for the defence acknowledged that endocarditis was a possible diagnosis to explain an illness of 6 weeks' duration with lethargy, fever and night sweats, and that administration of antibiotics may have clouded the presentation of endocarditis. Nevertheless, he wrote that, in spite of not being able to explain the mild elevation of the white cell and neutrophil counts, they were not due to infectious endocarditis.

He was unable to provide an alternative diagnosis to explain Dawn's illness. The microbiologist argued that endocarditis was excluded because the Duke criteria (see below) were not met. The microbiologist referred to literature about native valve endocarditis and mitral valve endocarditis, neither of which was relevant.

A cardiologist expert witness for the defence acknowledged that it was not possible to completely exclude endocarditis unless a definite other diagnosis was found. The cardiologist asserted that Dawn's symptoms may well have been due to cerebellar ischaemia, but he offered no explanation for the cause of the cerebellar ischaemia, other than infective endocarditis. He argued that even if endocarditis were the diagnosis, earlier treatment would not have altered the outcome.

A cardiologist expert witness for the plaintiff considered that it was always rational and appropriate to retain differential diagnoses such as endocarditis which are associated with significant morbidity and mortality until they can be safely excluded, and an alternative diagnosis is made. Earlier diagnosis and treatment would more likely than not have prevented Dawn's death.

The case is ongoing.

Discussion

Prosthetic valve endocarditis is potentially lethal. It is for this reason that endocarditis should be retained as a provisional diagnosis in a patient with a prosthetic heart valve who remains unwell for several weeks with fever, lethargy and night sweats. The Duke criteria for diagnosis of endocarditis are not a substitute for clinical judgment when no diagnosis other than endocarditis is established to explain the symptoms and signs. Guidelines and scoring systems are valuable clinical tools. They are based on the premise that all cases will fit the rules. This is a dangerous assumption for some conditions. This is not to diminish the importance of the tools or to denigrate those responsible for their formulation. It is simply a warning to think outside the box. While adherence to accepted guidelines may arguably be a good defence to a claim in negligence, it may not always be in a patient's best interest.

The major Duke criteria for endocarditis include 2 separate positive blood cultures with an organism likely to cause endocarditis and echocardiographic features typical of infection. If both major criteria are present, endocarditis is proved. In Dawn's case initial blood cultures in hospital were probably negative because of oral antibiotic therapy she had received prior to admission. No echocardiogram was obtained prior to cerebellar infarction.

It was probable that cerebellar infarction was due to embolisation of infective material from the aortic valve. This is likely to have accounted for the absence of transoesophageal echocardiographic evidence of a prosthetic valve vegetation following cerebellar infarction.

There are five minor Duke criteria for endocarditis including a predisposing heart condition or intravenous drug use, fever above 38°C, evidence of emboli, immunologic phenomena, microbiological evidence of infection, but not sufficient for a major Duke criterion, and echocardiographic findings that do not meet a Duke major criterion. If all minor criteria are fulfilled, endocarditis is proved.

Dawn had an underlying heart condition predisposing her to endocarditis. She presented with a history of fever and night sweats, although she was not febrile in hospital after receiving multiple courses of oral antibiotic therapy. She had cerebellar infarction, likely due to embolism. There was progressive elevation of CRP. There was progressive neutrophil leucocytosis. No echocardiogram was performed prior to cerebellar infarction. Endocarditis was not excluded.

Importantly, in Dawn's case, no diagnosis other than endocarditis was established to explain her illness.

When Dawn presented to hospital, Dr Anand noted that previous oral antibiotic therapy may cloud the presentation of endocarditis. He emphasised the need to consider endocarditis. Dr Anand discussed Dawn's illness with her usual cardiologist, Dr Subahdar. Dr Subahdar relied on the absence of elevation of CRP on admission to form his opinion that endocarditis was unlikely, and he declined to have Dawn admitted to hospital under his care. Dr Subahdar was consulted after Dawn became confused due to increased intracranial pressure following cerebellar infarction. Three hours before Dr Subahdar's review of Dawn on 27 May 2013 the CRP had risen above the upper limit of normal, yet Dr Subahdar irrationally maintained that the CRP was normal and stable.

Dawn was transferred to a referral centre for surgical decompression of her brain. The diagnosis at the referral centre was cerebellar infarction due to embolisation from the aortic valve. Surgical decompression of the brain and intravenous antibiotic therapy did not save Dawn's life.

If Dawn had received appropriate intravenous antibiotic therapy sooner than was the case, she may have survived.

Prosthetic valve endocarditis is usually lethal in the absence of explantation of the infected valve and replacement with a new prosthesis. It is often clinically valuable to discuss management of a patient such as Dawn at a heart team meeting comprising cardiologists, cardiothoracic surgeons, cardiothoracic anaesthetists and intensivists, in order to plan optimal therapy. The consensus opinion at such a meeting would likely have been that intravenous antibiotic therapy should be continued for 6 weeks, with specific advice from an infectious diseases physician. Elective prosthetic valve replacement could have been scheduled during this period.

In the absence of haemorrhagic transformation of cerebellar infarction, there was not a strong reason to omit prosthetic valve replacement during the period of intravenous antibiotic therapy. The potential risk of death associated with prosthetic valve endocarditis without replacement of the infected valve was likely greater than the potential risk of haemorrhagic stroke during anticoagulation for cardiopulmonary bypass to permit replacement of the infected prosthetic aortic valve.

Clinical Principles

This case illustrates the importance of retaining a potentially lethal differential diagnosis until such a diagnosis is excluded and replaced with a benign diagnosis. It also highlights the pitfalls of diagnostic and treatment algorithms. Dr Anand, emergency medicine specialist, recognised that endocarditis should not be excluded. Dr Subahdar, the cardiologist, too readily dismissed the diagnosis based on absence of elevation of CRP at the time, notwithstanding the fact that his patient had a prosthetic aortic valve and had been persistently unwell for several weeks with lethargy, fever and night sweats. Dr Subahdar ignored the facts that the CRP had been elevated prior to admission and that Dawn had received several courses of oral antibiotic therapy.

He declined to reconsider the diagnosis of endocarditis when Dawn had cerebellar infarction, based on the false notion that the CRP had not risen. If Dr Subahdar had kept an open mind in respect of the potential lethal diagnosis of endocarditis, he would not have overlooked the facts that the CRP was rising and that no diagnosis other than endocarditis had been made to explain Dawn's illness.

MOTHER KNOWS BEST

History

Aiden Maclean, aged 3 years, attended kindergarten. After lunch one day, he felt unwell and was collected by his mother, Morag, on the advice of the preschool staff. At about 16:30 h, Morag phoned the office of Dr Bruce Hunter, a general practitioner with 20 years of experience, and the regular doctor of all the Macleans, to make an appointment for urgent review before the office shut at 18:00 h. She was told that there were no appointments for that day and that Aiden could be seen the following morning.

The next day, Morag told Dr Hunter that for 24 hours Aiden had had headaches, listlessness, reluctance to walk, a sore leg, difficulty sleeping, loss of appetite, vomiting and an area of discolouration on the elbow. Dr Hunter noted that Aiden appeared subdued and quiet. He recorded a history of headache, vomiting and sore legs. He wrote that there was no diarrhoea. The temperature was 37.4°C, the abdomen was soft and there was no abnormality found in the ears, nose, throat or chest. There was no record of Aiden's hydration status or of any examination of the legs, or of the presence of a bruise on the elbow.

Dr Hunter concluded that Aiden was suffering from a viral infection and he was given supportive management.

The following day Aiden complained of a sore right foot and was unable to walk unassisted. Morag carried Aiden into the office of Dr Hunter. Aiden was obviously unwell. Dr Hunter noted the sore right foot, along with cellulitis and a rash on the great toe.

Dr Hunter discussed management with a general practitioner colleague in the practice. They agreed to send Aiden to a paediatrician for urgent review, but Aiden was not sent directly to hospital. The provisional diagnosis by the paediatrician was meningococcal septicaemia. Aiden was then sent straight to hospital.

On arriving at the hospital at 14:10 h Aiden's temperature was 39°C and amongst other findings there were two areas of purpura. The doctors instituted a septic work up. Blood, urine and spinal fluid were taken for culture and intravenous antibiotics were commenced. The CRP four hours later was 352 mg/L (reference <5 mg/L) and the ESR was 33 mm/h (reference <20 mm/h). Blood cultures grew *Staphylococcus aureus*, and an echocardiogram showed vegetations on the aortic valve, for which surgery was required.

LEGAL ISSUES

Aiden's family sued Dr Hunter in negligence for the delayed diagnosis of aortic valve endocarditis. They also sued him for nervous shock. Opinions were sought from independent general practitioners, cardiologists and infectious diseases physicians.

As is often the case, the experts' opinions depended on the set of assumptions given to them by the lawyers requesting a report. In that regard, the history as given by Morag differed in some respects from the history recorded by Dr Hunter. In particular, there was a dispute about the presence of a bruise on the elbow and a sore leg (rather than general aches).

The plaintiff's expert was also critical of the failure of the receptionist to seek the advice of one of the general practitioners in the practice to ascertain whether Aiden required urgent review or referral to the local hospital emergency department.

The defendant also relied on expert cardiology and infectious diseases opinion that, even with earlier diagnosis, the aortic valve would still have required surgery.

The case is ongoing.

DISCUSSION

Morag endeavoured to make an appointment for urgent review on the day Aiden became unwell. Although Dr Hunter worked in a practice with other doctors, no appointment was offered for review by any of the doctors that day, and Morag was not advised to take Aiden to hospital.

It is almost axiomatic in medical practice that a mother knows better than anyone else when her child is ill. It is also well understood that the clinical condition of a young child may deteriorate rapidly. Young children are often unable to provide an accurate history; they need to rely on their parents, which is, in a majority of cases, the mother.

If it had been recognised on day one that Aiden was unwell, he would likely have been admitted to hospital for urgent investigation and management. His illness would have been treated earlier than was the case, and he may have avoided aortic valve surgery. Many receptionists in general practices are qualified nurses. Many practices also engage nurse practitioners. It is not known whether that was the case at Dr Hunter's practice. A receptionist who is given a triage role in a general practice is often placed in a difficult position. The general practitioners in the practice must ensure that a receptionist is properly instructed as to when a call should be put through to one of the doctors. A receptionist cannot be relied upon in all cases to ask the right questions of parents or to recognise risky situations.

When Aiden was eventually reviewed the next day, Dr Hunter failed to explore all the clinical features Morag had described, and failed to examine Aiden thoroughly. If Dr Hunter had performed a more comprehensive examination he would likely have concluded that Aiden needed investigation in hospital. A viral infection was unlikely to be responsible for all Aiden's symptoms and signs, including purpura or unilateral foot pain.

When Aiden was unable to walk unassisted and was brought back to Dr Hunter two days after his symptoms commenced, Dr Hunter consulted a colleague in his practice, and they arranged urgent review by a paediatrician.

Sending Aiden from Dr Hunter's office to see a paediatrician wasted valuable time. A better approach would have been to discuss the matter with the paediatric registrar at the local paediatric referral hospital. Immediate hospital admission would have been advised. Whether aortic valve surgery could have been avoided at this late stage is moot.

Dr Hunter had more than 20 years of experience as a general practitioner. One of the cardinal skills of a general practitioner is to recognise when a child is ill. On day two Aiden had 24 hours of fever, a leg sufficiently painful that he was unwilling to walk, a history of vomiting, lethargy and a rash on both the foot and an elbow.

Various emergency drugs, including penicillin, are available free of charge to general practitioners to be used as necessary. Did this practice keep such a supply, and if not, why not?

Dr Hunter had three options. The first was to discuss the matter urgently with the paediatric registrar on call at the referral hospital; the second was to administer penicillin urgently in the belief that Aiden had septicaemia, probably meningococcal; and the third was to refer Aiden to a paediatrician in his office.

Of those three options, referral to a paediatrician was the least appropriate, because the possibility of systemic bacterial infection requires immediate investigation and treatment.

Clinical Principles

It is a foolhardy doctor, or doctor's receptionist, who refuses a request from a concerned mother of a young child with an acute illness for the child to be seen that day.

Septicaemia is usually rapidly progressive. The constellation of Aiden's symptoms and signs should have prompted immediate hospital admission, on the basis of probable systemic bacterial infection. The fact that Aiden was only 3 years old and may not have been able to articulate all his symptoms underlined the urgency of the situation.

The notation that Aiden appeared to be subdued and quiet should have alerted Dr Hunter to the fact that Aiden was severely unwell. This was particularly pertinent as Aiden was an existing patient of Dr Hunter.

NECROTISING FASCIITIS

In this chapter we discuss three cases of necrotising fasciitis. This is a potentially lethal infection often associated with tissue loss. The keys to management are early recognition of the diagnosis and intensive intravenous antibiotic therapy. Surgery is often required.

ONE LAST CRY FOR HELP

HISTORY

Barbara Napaljarri was a 33-year-old indigenous woman. She lived in a remote mixed-race community of 3000 people where there was a twenty-bed hospital. She had been an enthusiastic student, and had been schooled in the local community until age 13. Her written and oral communication was that expected of her level of schooling. In her late teens she obtained a position in the local hospital as a nurse's aide. Barbara performed satisfactorily until she developed a liking for alcohol and illicit substances. Morphine was her favourite, but she would happily use whatever else she could acquire, including marijuana and amphetamines.

Her employment at the hospital was terminated, after which she presented to the hospital on frequent occasions, usually about once every seven to ten days, over many years complaining of severe abdominal pain that was only relieved by an injection of morphine. Simple measures such as intravenous fluids, bed rest and antiemetics were ineffective. One of her habits on admission was to raid the linen supply and grab a collection of towels. She would then have very frequent showers, often every half hour or so.

If she did not receive the narcotic she craved she would be loud, destructive and rolling in pain maybe for a day or so until the medical staff gave in and administered morphine. Soon after each injection the pain would suddenly resolve, after which she would self-discharge.

She had been referred to a regional hospital for investigation of her symptoms, but an organic reason could not be demonstrated.

One day Barbara presented to the emergency department with an area of spreading cellulitis on her back, for which she was admitted and treated with intravenous antibiotics. She complained bitterly to Dr Andrew O'Mara, whom she had encountered before, that she had severe pain. Dr O'Mara presumed that Barbara was simply craving morphine, as well as coincidentally having cellulitis. He refused to accept that Barbara's pain was genuine. It appeared to be out of proportion to the severity of the cellulitis he observed. Accordingly, he concluded her requests for narcotic analgesia had nothing to do with her presenting illness. Twenty-four hours later she was febrile and toxic. Dr O'Mara sought advice from the referral hospital, to which Barbara was airlifted as a matter of urgency.

She died the following day of necrotising fasciitis and septic shock.

Barbara had been a respected member of the local community particularly as she was articulate in her own language and could read and write well in English. It was suspected that Barbara was able to supply prohibited substances, at a price, to those who desired such.

Soon after it was known that Barbara had died there was great unrest among the indigenous community and Dr O'Mara was blamed for her death. It was determined that 'pay back' would take place. The police were called. They instructed Dr O'Mara to pack his bags immediately. They drove him to a safe-house, and escorted him to a plane early the next morning. Dr O'Mara never returned.

Legal Issues

The superintendent of the referral hospital was not willing to supply a death certificate. Since Barbara's death was sudden, there was a coronial inquiry. It was found that Barbara had died because of fulminant necrotising fasciitis despite appropriate antibiotic therapy. Even if Dr O'Mara had appreciated the urgency of the situation, Barbara would still have died. Civil proceedings were not initiated.

Discussion

This case highlights the need for continuity of care, but also the dangers of assuming all complaints of a particular symptom such as pain will always be due to the same thing or will always be due to a non-organic cause.

There will always be risks of litigation in remote communities when medical practitioners change on a frequent basis. This will continue to be the case wherever staff turnover is high. Some remote communities do not have a permanent doctor and need to rely on a series of itinerant locums. The plausible drug seeking patient is likely to find such doctors an easy target for their well-rehearsed stories, where there may be a tendency to take the easy way out and provide them with what they seek. Another factor that may affect management sometimes is that locum nurses are not familiar with their patients. This was probably not relevant in Barbara's case because she had a new problem of necrotising fasciitis.

In this case Dr O'Mara knew Barbara and had seen her before. He was familiar with her demands for narcotics. He may well have been blind-sided by this familiarity, thinking that this was another of Barbara's demands for morphine without an organic indication. He should have considered at least the possibility that Barbara's complaint of pain was related to her presenting illness before excluding it as being part and parcel of her usual drug-seeking behaviour. Necrotising fasciitis may be associated with cellulitis. One of its characteristic features is pain disproportionate to the observed infection. Dr

O'Mara missed an opportunity to transfer Barbara for potentially life-saving treatment when he closed his mind to an organic basis to her complaints of pain.

Pay back is a traditional punishment when an indigenous community believes that a great wrong has been committed, and is similar to the biblical 'eye for an eye and a tooth for a tooth'. Anyone who has worked in such remote communities for long enough would have encountered such a threat, usually from an alcohol-affected patient who does not get what he or she perceives is needed and what the doctor is unwilling to supply. Such a threat can usually be ignored; however not in this case.

One working in a remote community sometimes encounters other indigenous cultural behaviours. A woman with a chest infection had been an in-patient for five days at the hospital and was well enough to go home. She refused to be discharged until a witchetty grub was brought to her. A friend arrived with a grub in a box filled with straw. The patient examined the grub twice a day and after three days the grub had died whereupon the patient swallowed the grub and then, believing that she was cured, left the hospital.

Another woman had been an inpatient for some days because of diverticulitis and was ready for discharge. That did not appeal to her and she asked for the local medicine-man. Thirty-six hours later an indigenous man, unknown to anyone at the hospital, arrived and spent one hour with the patient in a closed room. After this healing process the patient left the hospital.

These last two patients allow one to understand the deeply held views of some who do not have a cultural history of western medicine. The medicine man may well have been a well-respected healer of indigenous patients for many years, maybe millennia, and the treatment by antibiotics in the hospital was merely incidental to the patient's recovery. The witchetty grub may have been also used for many years for healing and the hospital management was simply a coincidence in the view of the patient.

This allows one to reflect on the healing that some patients experience at the hands of their doctor with whom the patient has great confidence, even though the medical practitioner at a particular consultation offers little more than reassurance. Drug-seeking behaviours are frustrating and difficult to differentiate from organic illness. This does not mean attempts to distinguish between the two should be minimised. By jumping to conclusions about Barbara, Dr O'Mara neither inspired confidence nor gave reassurance when it was required.

Clinical Principles

Whenever a patient presents complaining of pain, it is important to evaluate the symptoms and signs and to exclude potentially serious pathology. Barbara had evidence of severe sepsis when she presented to the local hospital for the last time, and she was treated with antibiotics. Her rapid clinical decline could not have been predicted, and earlier transfer to the referral centre may not have altered the outcome. Her pain, however, appeared inconsistent with the severity of her cellulitis. Rather than being fobbed off as drug-seeking behaviour, consideration of an underlying more serious infection should have occurred.

SEVERE PAIN AFTER EXCISION OF A SMALL SKIN LESION

HISTORY

Beryl Dooley, aged 65, had been feeling unwell with fevers and night sweats for a month prior to seeing Dr Basil Brown. During this month a small lesion appeared on her anterior chest, oozing blood. Dr Brown, who considered this to be a pyogenic granuloma, suggested that it be removed, to which Beryl agreed. The lesion was removed under local anaesthesia and Beryl returned home.

Beryl phoned Dr Brown later that day complaining of very severe pain. He prescribed paracetamol. Four hours later she again phoned Dr Brown, because of persistent and increasing pain. He advised her to take paracetamol 500 mg with codeine 30 mg even though Beryl had told him that codeine made her vomit. Ten hours later she presented to the local hospital where the diagnosis of necrotising fasciitis was made. Despite large doses of appropriate intravenous antibiotics, Beryl required bilateral mastectomies and a lengthy period in intensive care.

LEGAL ISSUES

Beryl sought compensation for the consequences of delayed diagnosis of necrotising fasciitis. She relied on the opinion of a general practitioner expert who considered Beryl should have been asked to return for review when she complained of worsening pain. It was unsafe for Dr Brown to assume the pain was normal post-procedure discomfort without first ruling out an infection, including a severe infection.

Divergent opinions were also obtained by both parties from infectious diseases physicians about whether prompt referral to hospital for antibiotic therapy would have avoided Beryl's pain and disfigurement.

The matter settled at mediation.

DISCUSSION

Dr Brown was obviously unaware of the implication of pain greatly in excess of what one would have clinically expected after a minor surgical procedure. This feature suggested necrotising fasciitis.

The condition requires both intensive antibiotic therapy and urgent surgical debridement. Patients with necrotising fasciitis have a poor prognosis. Without rapid and effective therapy the mortality rate is ~30%.

General practitioners need to understand the limits of their expertise when performing procedures. They may be sufficiently or even superbly skillful, but expertise also encompasses knowledge of risks and their treatment.

Clinical Principles

Anyone performing surgical procedures, even minor ones, needs to know about necrotising fasciitis and the need for rapid management. Its cardinal feature is the presence of pain greatly in excess of what one would expect following a simple infection or a simple surgical procedure.

RIGORS AND SCROTAL PAIN

History

Brian Schipp was holidaying overseas when he had an acute coronary syndrome requiring coronary artery stenting. He had a previous history of both coronary artery disease and urethral obstruction with the latter needing dilation and urethral catheterisation. Attempts to introduce a catheter whilst overseas were unsuccessful and he returned home with a suprapubic catheter, accompanied by a medical escort.

On arriving home he attended a urologist where unsuccessful attempts were made to introduce a urethral catheter. At urethroscopy it was not possible to completely relieve the stricture, and the suprapubic catheter remained in situ. During the procedure gentamicin 240 mg was administered. Brian was discharged home for review by the urologist four weeks later.

The following day Brian began to feel unwell and experienced rigors. Several days later he attended his general practitioner, Dr Carol Crawford, with generalised malaise and aches, and very painful swollen testicles. Dr Crawford examined him briefly and prescribed norfloxacin. She advised Brian to attend the hospital if he did not improve.

After several further days Brian presented himself back to the urological centre, where necrotising fasciitis (Fournier's gangrene) was diagnosed. The infection caused necrosis and sloughing of the anterior scrotum. Brian remained in hospital for several months, during which time he required surgery and prolonged intravenous antibiotic therapy.

Legal Issues

Brian sued Dr Crawford for damages in negligence for the consequences of delayed diagnosis and treatment of necrotising fasciitis. Based on expert general practitioner evidence, Brian argued that contact with or referral back to the urologist should have taken place when he presented with general malaise, rigors and an exceedingly painful, swollen scrotum. The symptoms and signs were suggestive of a serious local and systemic infection.

As with the prior cases, there was a dispute between the causation experts (infectious diseases physicians and urologists) as to whether earlier referral would have halted progression of the necrotising fasciitis and horrendous outcome.

The case settled at mediation.

Discussion

Brian had unsuccessful surgical treatment for urethral stricture, overseas and in Australia. He had a suprapubic catheter and was at increased risk for infection. It is not known exactly when necrotising fasciitis commenced. Nevertheless it would have been appropriate, if not essential, for Dr Crawford to contact the urologist as soon as Brian was unwell. The urologist could then have consulted an expert in infectious diseases to ensure that Brian was investigated immediately and was prescribed appropriate aggressive intravenous antibiotic therapy. This may have arrested the progression of necrotising fasciitis.

Therapeutic Guidelines (a well recognised Australian reference source) suggests the combination of ampicillin and gentamicin for severe pelvic infection. Brian received gentamicin at the time of urethroscopy, and norfloxacin when he had rigors and tender swollen testicles. He was not admitted immediately to hospital when there was evidence of severe infection because his general practitioner assumed management of his condition in circumstances where specialist input was required from Brian's urologist.

Clinical Principles

Necrotising fasciitis is a potentially lethal and disfiguring infection. While unusual, it needs to be on the diagnostic radar when a patient's symptoms, especially pain, are out of proportion to observable signs or when progression of a local infection appears unusually rapid. Combination intravenous antibiotic therapy is always required. Tissue loss is common, and surgery is often indicated to limit the spread of infection.

SORE WRIST

History

Tom Wood, a 37-year-old house painter, was seated in his stationary car one day in 2000, when a truck travelling at ~100 km/hr struck his vehicle from behind. Tom was dazed but did not lose consciousness. He returned home unaided, and later on experienced severe pain and tenderness in many areas of the body, including his right wrist.

When he attended the local hospital the following day, there was tenderness in the neck muscles and in muscles and joints elsewhere, due to the whiplash injury. X-rays revealed four fractured ribs, and a right scaphoid fracture. Tom was referred to his usual general practitioner, Dr Bill Taniane, for review. Dr Taniane did not follow-up the scaphoid fracture at the time.

Several months elapsed before Tom regained reasonable function overall. The whiplash neck injury troubled him for longer. He required regular analgesia and suffered from reactive depression, particularly as he was unable to work.

The following year he suffered an injury to his right thumb when he fell whilst using a power saw to chop firewood. Examination at the local hospital demonstrated a deep laceration of the right thumb, involving the distal phalanx, which was shattered, and almost severed. Even though it was unlikely that simple laceration repair would be sufficient to ensure an optimal functional result, primary wound repair was performed, without referral to a specialist hand surgeon. Tom returned home later that day with a prescription for oral flucloxacillin, to be managed by Dr Taniane.

Tom complained of pain at the site of the old scaphoid fracture. Dr Taniane ordered an x-ray of the right hand. This showed a fine lucent line extending through the proximal pole of the scaphoid. The radiologist recommended a review x-ray one week later. Although Dr Taniane's records referred to the need for a follow-up x-ray, there was no evidence that this review x-ray was requested or performed. Dr Taniane did not provide further prescriptions for antibiotics, and did not record details of history or physical findings.

A month after the accident, Dr Taniane noted wrist pain but recorded no other information. Tom saw Dr Taniane seven times during the following four months, for pain relief and dressings. Dr Taniane ultimately referred Tom to a consultant general surgeon.

Tom told the surgeon that he had constant unrelenting right thumb pain with marked hypersensitivity. Sutures from the repair four months previously were still in situ. Both the metacarpophalangeal and interphalangeal joints were very stiff. The surgeon diagnosed reflex sympathetic dystrophy.

X-rays showed marked disuse osteoporosis in the thumb, with a distal phalanx comminuted fracture. A bone scan demonstrated low-grade periarticular uptake at the metacarpophalangeal and interphalangeal joints, compatible with reflex sympathetic dystrophy. There was also increased tracer uptake at the proximal pole of the right scaphoid, indicating either a fracture or avascular necrosis. Dr Taniane did not inform the surgeon of any previous x-rays or findings of a possible scaphoid fracture.

The fracture of the distal phalangeal bone remained ununited, with bone resorption. Tom subsequently saw two orthopaedic surgeons, both of whom agreed that amputation at the level of the interphalangeal joint was indicated, particularly as the distal stump appeared to be nonviable. There was a suggestion of osteomyelitis in the distal phalanx. Both the erythrocyte sedimentation rate (ESR) and the CRP level were normal, indicating that osteomyelitis was unlikely. The amputation took place and this was uneventful.

There continued to be radiological evidence of the possibility of either infection or fracture in the scaphoid. Avascular necrosis could not be excluded. It was at this time that the latter orthopaedic surgeon, this being the fourth medical practitioner to see Tom since the motor vehicle accident, turned his attention to the scaphoid region, in addition to the fractured phalanx.

Tom told the second orthopaedic surgeon that since the car accident four years previously, he had suffered constant pain in the right wrist and that he had been unable to use the wrist as before because of soreness and stiffness. All of the previous x-rays were then reviewed. One taken two years following the car accident showed an undisplaced fracture in the middle of the scaphoid. A bone scan after this x-ray demonstrated an abnormality in the proximal pole of the scaphoid.

The x-rays taken three years after the car accident had clearly shown the scaphoid fracture. Four years after the car accident, an x-ray showed an ununited fracture of the proximal pole of the scaphoid with bone resorption and a large cystic lesion.

Tom ultimately proceeded to internal fixation and bone grafting, followed by cast immobilisation for eight weeks. Progress x-rays six months following the graft showed very slow healing with some features of avascular necrosis without evidence of fracture union. The orthopaedic surgeon referred Tom to a hand surgeon to consider the possibility of a vascular graft. The hand surgeon did not recommend a further operative procedure because of the very significant degree of stiffness in the wrist joint. She was also concerned about the medicolegal risk if further surgery did not produce the desired result.

At six years following the car accident, and four years following the thumb laceration, x-rays revealed almost complete union of the scaphoid fracture.

The stump of the thumb remained sore, cold and hypersensitive to touch. The wrist, which was a greater problem than the thumb, remained sore, stiff and weak. The whole hand remained somewhat cold. The various consultants who considered his position believed that his prognosis for long-term work was poor.

Tom returned to painting part-time. He avoided using a brush if possible, and preferred to use a roller. It remains to be seen whether he will be able to continue working.

Legal Issues

Tom sought compensation for physical disability and psychological stress associated with inadequate care following the motor vehicle accident, and following the laceration. The case was settled at mediation.

Discussion

An array of issues arises, with the first being the rational use of antibiotics following the lacerated finger. Tom was prescribed only one course of antibiotics, despite the risk of developing osteomyelitis. As it happened, osteomyelitis did not develop.

Next, Dr Taniane's notes were brief and unhelpful. The initial x-ray indicated a fracture of the scaphoid, which should not have been ignored. Earlier effective management of the scaphoid fracture may well have allowed healing without long-term morbid sequelae.

The sutures ought not to have been left in the wound for four months after the emergency department presentation, until Tom was referred to the general surgeon.

It is of interest that both the general surgeon and the orthopaedic surgeons were not initially aware of the scaphoid fracture because Dr Taniane did not inform them that an x-ray of the scaphoid had been taken. Tom had reflex sympathetic dystrophy and it was thought initially that pain in the hand was caused by this (since reflex sympathetic dystrophy may cause generalised pain in the region). Pain related to the scaphoid fracture was unrecognised at first.

The hand surgeon, who was aware of the medicolegal implications, decided not to become involved. She believed that success with surgery was unlikely. There was in her mind the question of the origin of the scaphoid fracture. Did the fracture occur at the time of the car accident, or did it occur when he fell while chopping firewood? Based on the history, it was more likely that the scaphoid fracture was caused by the accident in 2000, since Tom had complained of wrist pain ever since then.

When only one of the small bones of the wrist is injured it is almost always the scaphoid, and there is a phylogenetic reason for this. The scaphoid, which is the largest of the carpal bones, is located at the base of the wrist. It allows movement of the adjacent bones, and is perfectly able to last the life of its owner if it is not injured. It is sometimes described as the cornerstone of the wrist; but it is a potentially unreliable cornerstone.

Its first deficiency is its configuration. The scaphoid is shaped somewhat like a canoe (in Greek scaphoides means boat-like), the result of fusion of two bones, the primitive scaphoid and the os centrale of lower hominoids. This fusion may have arisen when hominoids became knuckle walkers as a prelude to bipedalism, with the fused bones increasing midcarpal stability. The primitive scaphoid and the os centrale together form the modern scaphoid.

The second deficiency is the need for this irregularly shaped bone to articulate with no fewer than five other bones, each adding movement stress, to the inherent instability of the scaphoid due to its geometry.

The third deficiency is related to blood supply. The primitive scaphoid and the os centrale each have their own blood supply. At the point of fusion, there is watershed perfusion. This is where non-union of a fracture is likely to occur.

These anatomical features explain why the scaphoid rather than the other seven carpal bones is the one usually fractured in a fall onto the wrist. Because of its relation to other wrist bones, scaphoid fracture commonly causes long-term wrist dysfunction, pain and stiffness. A better understanding of anatomy may have helped Dr Taniane to diagnose Tom's problem.

Clinical Principles

This case is an example of a communication problem. Dr Taniane knew about a probable scaphoid fracture soon after the thumb injury, but neither managed this problem nor alerted the surgeons to it. When the general surgeon saw Tom with pain in the hand, he assumed the pain was entirely due to reflex sympathetic dystrophy. This was not the case.

Although the scaphoid problem rested mainly on Dr Taniane's lack of communication, it is true that the surgeon could have taken a more adequate history. If it had been noted that hand pain had been present since the car accident, the scaphoid fracture would likely have been managed sooner.

The failure to remove the sutures (inadequate physical examination) and the lack of adequate medical records indicated a lack of diligence on Dr Taniane's part.

This case is also an example of failure to appreciate the significance of radiological findings. If Dr Taniane had registered the presence of a scaphoid fracture on x-rays after the motor vehicle accident, earlier intervention may have improved the outcome.

INGESTION OF A CAUSTIC SOLUTION

HISTORY

On 2 May 2016, Margaret Buchanan dropped her three-year-old daughter, Maddie, at her parents' house on the way to work. Margaret's parents were in their seventies. They regularly looked after Maddie so that Margaret could work part-time at the local school as a relief teacher. At about 11:00 h on 2 May 2016, Maddie's grandmother, Heather, was startled by Maddie's sudden screaming and crying. Heather stopped preparing morning tea to attend to her granddaughter.

Her granddaughter was near the water cooler in the kitchen. She was drooling, her lips were swollen and when Maddie spoke she had a hoarse voice. Heather was worried by Maddie's condition. She yelled out to her husband, Ron, to attend. He told Heather that he had recently cleaned the water cooler but had otherwise not seen Maddie access anything from cupboards or the pantry. Neither had Heather. Heather telephoned Margaret on her mobile phone and advised her that she and Ron were taking Maddie to the local emergency department because she looked as though she was very ill.

By the time Maddie presented to the emergency department, she was vomiting and had stridor. A senior emergency department doctor immediately saw her. He noted swollen lips, oropharyngeal oedema, stridor, uncontrollable drooling and a hoarse voice. He was concerned about anaphylaxis to an unknown agent and administered adrenaline and dexamethasone. After administration of these medications, Maddie still vomited, still had stridor and her lips and mouth remained swollen. Her mother, Margaret, arrived soon after.

The emergency specialist obtained a history of events at Heather and Ron's house. He was told that Maddie had had no access to any poisons or other substances, but had been near the water cooler at the time she suddenly started screaming and crying. Ron told the doctor that he had used caustic soda to clean the water cooler, but was sure that he had washed it out of the system.

The consultant paediatrician at the hospital was asked to review Maddie. On examination, the paediatrician noted swelling of the oropharynx, including inflammation of the tonsils with possible slough. A chest x-ray was performed, which demonstrated mild prominence of the perihilar bronchovascular markings consistent with an inflammatory or a viral infective response. The paediatrician considered the differential diagnoses to be ingestion of a foreign body, ingestion of a toxic compound, trauma to the oropharynx or an anaphylactic reaction. Because the local hospital did not have the services and facilities to manage some of these conditions, she arranged urgent transfer to a tertiary children's hospital. She advised, in the referring letter and on the telephone to the paediatric emergency department, that one of the differential diagnoses was caustic ingestion.

When Maddie arrived at the paediatric emergency department at the tertiary hospital, she was seen by one of the junior emergency medical staff, who considered the possibility of acute tonsillitis, but thought that caustic ingestion needed to be excluded, especially as the referring paediatrician had thought it to be a possible cause. The doctor requested the ear, nose and throat (ENT) team to review Maddie.

The ENT registrar, Dr Nigella Crowhurst, subsequently examined Maddie in the emergency department. She noticed swelling of the oropharynx and lips together with inflammation of the tonsils, uvula and soft palate with associated slough. Dr Crowhurst was particularly impressed by the inflamed appearance of the tonsils and what she thought was some type of exudate on their surface. She reassured Margaret and her parents that Maddie had an infection, which would come under control with antibiotics. Maddie was kept overnight for observation and administered intravenous antibiotics. She continued to vomit, refused food and water and continually drooled. The next day, despite Margaret's protestations, Maddie was discharged for follow-up in one week's time in the ENT outpatient department of the hospital. She was prescribed an antibiotic liquid. The junior emergency doctor thought Maddie should be investigated further, but nonetheless followed Dr Crowhurst's decision. Margaret complained that Maddie was unwell and that it did not seem to be tonsillitis to her, having experienced it herself and noting the symptoms one of her other children had when he had acute tonsillitis.

Maddie was taken to the ENT outpatient department one week after discharge. There, she was again seen by Dr Crowhurst. In the week following discharge, Maddie had decreased oral intake, vomiting and was generally unwell. Dr Crowhurst examined Maddie's pharynx and noted that there was still inflammation and swelling. She prescribed further antibiotics and advised Maddie's mother that it would settle in time. She was advised to return in two weeks for a check up.

Maddie continued to be unwell after the ENT review. She had bouts of vomiting frothy mucus, gagging, abdominal pain, decreased oral intake, drooling and a husky voice. On 4 June 2016, Margaret took her daughter to the emergency department at the local hospital. She was hesitant about returning to the tertiary children's hospital because she felt that she had not been listened to. Maddie was seen in the emergency department and then again by the paediatrician who had examined her on 2 May 2016. The paediatrician obtained a history of markedly reduced eating, apart from small amounts of icecream, vomiting, gagging, hoarseness, weight loss and drooling. The paediatrician thought there was likely to be oesophageal obstruction. She ordered a lateral chest x-ray, took throat swabs and inserted an intravenous line. The throat swabs were negative. The lateral x-ray demonstrated narrowing of the middle third of the oesophagus. Maddie was referred to a different tertiary children's hospital for investigation and treatment of obstruction of the oesophagus.

On 5 June 2016, Maddie was admitted to the children's hospital, and underwent a barium swallow. This demonstrated a stricture of the oesophagus. A paediatric surgeon was asked to review Maddie. He recommended an urgent laryngobronchoscopy and oesophagoscopy. At operation, the surgeon found a 12 cm oesophageal stricture in the middle third of the oesophagus. There were two other smaller strictures. Maddie proceeded to balloon dilation. She subsequently underwent multiple oesophageal dilations (in excess of 12), a fundoplication and a percutaneous endoscopic gastrostomy (PEG) to assist with feeding. Her future is uncertain.

Legal Issues

In 2018, Margaret commenced proceedings against the entity responsible for the tertiary children's hospital Maddie presented to on 2 May 2016. She brought the proceedings on Maddie's behalf as her tutor (because Maddie was a minor) and on her own behalf for nervous shock as a result of experiencing Maddie's injuries and disabilities. Maddie's husband, Howard, also brought a claim for nervous shock.

The case was supported by the opinions of a paediatric gastroenterologist, an ear nose and throat surgeon and an emergency specialist. All accepted that an infective process was a reasonable diagnosis to have been considered by staff at the children's hospital. They also considered that a differential diagnosis of anaphylaxis was reasonable initially, but not later when Maddie failed to respond to adrenaline and dexamethasone. The experts maintained that ingestion of a caustic compound ought to have been a differential diagnosis and investigated appropriately to confirm or exclude it. They noted that the paediatrician from the referring hospital had considered caustic ingestion as a possible cause of Maddie's symptoms and signs. It was one of the reasons Maddie was referred to a tertiary hospital on an urgent basis. The experts considered that the absence of a clear history of ingesting a poison or caustic compound was not determinative of the likely cause of Maddie's complaints. They noted that many childhood poisoning cases lack a clear history or even a denial of access to a poison. In Maddie's case, a reasonable suspicion was raised about the water cooler and its recent cleaning by Maddie's grandfather. Cleaning agents are generally caustic and represent a ready source of tissue injury with ingestion.

The emergency specialist and the ear nose and throat surgeon were critical of the diagnosis of acute tonsillitis. This is because tonsillitis was unlikely to be responsible for drooling, swollen lips, stridor or persistent vomiting (in the absence of a systemic infection). In addition, the history of the *sudden* onset of severe symptoms made acute tonsillitis most unlikely. The absence of a response to dexamethasone and adrenaline pointed away from a severe allergic reaction. In the circumstances, they considered that a paediatric gastroenterologist should have been asked to see Maddie. The pH of Maddie's saliva should also have been tested.

The paediatric gastroenterologist was of the opinion that the only way to diagnose caustic ingestion definitively was by gastroscopy or oesophagoscopy. While this is an unpleasant procedure and requires anaesthesia, it was essential for diagnosis.

In hindsight, there was no dispute that Maddie had ingested a caustic compound used for cleaning the water cooler. Her grandfather ultimately provided the bottle of caustic soda to staff at the second tertiary children's hospital. Thus, if a gastroscopy had been performed on or soon after 2 May 2016, oesophageal injury would have been demonstrated. In the circumstances, Maddie would then have been treated with antibiotics, proton pump inhibitors, corticosteroids and nil by mouth. She would have maintained adequate nutrition, would not have had repeated vomiting with acid refluxing into the oesophagus, would not have suffered trauma from swallowing food and would have been regularly monitored.

The dispute in the case was whether this treatment would have materially affected Maddie's outcome. While such treatment is recommended in cases of caustic ingestion, experts relied on by the defendant indicated that there is little persuasive epidemiological evidence proving the benefits of these measures. In addition, it was argued that all of the damage was done at the outset so that multiple and severe stricture formation was always going to occur even with earlier diagnosis and treatment.

While the care at the first tertiary referral hospital was arguably unsatisfactory, the defendant might not be found negligent because the breach of its duty of care may not be causally related to the outcome. If this occurs, then the staff at the hospital may not learn anything from the way they treated Maddie. Indeed, they may think their approach was vindicated.

The matter is ongoing.

Discussion

This case highlights two important aspects of medical care. The first is that parents are more likely to know whether their children are ill or even whether a proffered explanation by a doctor is reasonable. As we have repeatedly pointed out, if the history is good enough, a parent will generally lead a doctor to the correct diagnosis of their child's problem. Margaret was adamant that acute tonsillitis could not explain all of Maddie's problems. She intuitively knew something was wrong. She repeated her concerns to Dr Crowhurst at the ENT outpatient review seven days after discharge. She was again met with a brickbat.

The second point is the problem of communication between junior and senior staff in a hospital setting. Maddie was never seen by a consultant ENT surgeon at the time of her presentation or indeed at follow up. A senior emergency doctor never saw her. She was not seen by any member of the paediatric gastroenterology staff. In contrast, when Maddie was taken by her grandparents to the local emergency department, she was seen by both a senior emergency department specialist and the consultant paediatrician. The consultant paediatrician formed a reasonable list of differential diagnoses including caustic ingestion. The outcome may have been different if the junior emergency department doctor at the tertiary children's hospital had communicated to a senior practitioner in the emergency department or in the ENT team. Instead, he deferred to the ENT registrar as being more senior and with specialised knowledge about tonsillitis. This communication problem is known as an authority gradient. It represents an obstacle to effective communication when there is an actual or perceived hierarchy in authority or expertise. In this case, it meant that the junior emergency doctor was reluctant to communicate to senior staff, especially when it involved challenging the opinion of a more senior practitioner. (1)

Clinical Principles

Childhood poisoning is responsible for a significant number of presentations to paediatric emergency departments. Children have potential access to toxic, poisonous or caustic compounds in a house. Not all houses are poison-proof even when effective measures are thought to have been taken by a family. Grandparents may not be as alert to the problem as children's parents. Ingestion of a poison, including a caustic compound, should be suspected in all circumstances where there is a *sudden* onset of abnormal symptoms and signs, even without a clear history of access. Sometimes, it is necessary for junior medical staff to challenge the opinions of more senior staff. Patient safety should always be put ahead of personal feelings of embarrassment, anxiety about incurring the wrath of a senior consultant or fear of being perceived as a fool.

Reference

Cosby, K.S., Croskerry, P., 2004. Profiles in patient safety: authority gradients in medical error. Acad. Emerg. Med. 11 (12), 1341–1345.

HAEMOPTYSIS

History

Gregory Merton, aged 42, was a fit man, who enjoyed running half-marathons. In 2015 he travelled to Asia with his family for a three-week holiday after which he travelled alone to the USA via London on business. The itinerary from Asia to London to North America and back to Australia occupied 10 days. Because they were visiting Asia, all of the family had been vaccinated prior to their departure by their general practitioner, Dr Cameron Williams.

The return journey to Australia from the USA in economy class had been tiring on a crowded flight. Gregory arrived home with a sore throat and visited Dr Williams the next day. The brief medical record referred to a temperature of 37°C, clear chest, red throat, tonsils not enlarged, and no pus on tonsils. Dr Williams prescribed amoxicillin 500 mg tds.

The next week Dr Williams saw Gregory because he had coughed small amounts of blood (haemoptysis) on two occasions the previous day. Gregory said that he had stopped smoking 20 years previously. The chest was clear with good air entry. Dr Williams ordered a chest x-ray that did not demonstrate any abnormality. Although the radiologist suggested a CT scan, Dr Williams did not order one.

Two months later Dr Williams recorded that Gregory had postviral labyrinthitis. A fortnight after this, he recorded findings identical to those at the consultation when Gregory had reported coughing blood. Dr Williams made no diagnosis. He prescribed fluticasone propionate with salmeterol xinafoate by inhaler. These agents had been prescribed previously, probably without benefit.

Gregory returned to Dr Williams the next week with malaise and dyspnoea. Dr Williams suggested a blood test and asked Gregory to return if his symptoms worsened. Dr Williams made no diagnosis and Gregory did not improve.

At the next visit a few days later Dr Williams diagnosed "pneumonia-atypical", requested a second chest x-ray, and prescribed roxithromycin, amoxicillin and clavulanic acid. Dr Williams wrote on the x-ray request, "persistent shortness of breath and two episodes of haemoptysis in the past 10 weeks". The radiologist reported multiple opacities throughout the left lung, possibly indicating pneumonic consolidation in the left upper and lower lobes.

Three days later Dr Williams contacted Gregory's home to arrange a repeat chest x-ray the following month. He learned Gregory had passed away in hospital on the previous day with DVT in the right leg, and multiple pulmonary emboli.

Legal Issues

Gregory died because of an undiagnosed pulmonary embolism. His widow took legal action against Dr Williams, because death was avoidable. The case is ongoing.

Discussion

Gregory's unfortunate story raises many issues. He had returned from long-haul air travel and attended his usual general practitioner with respiratory symptoms the day following his return. Dr Williams was well aware of the air travel, as he had vaccinated the whole family prior to the travel.

Soon after the initial consultation Gregory returned with a history of coughing blood. For a traveller, this is the ultimate red flag. Dr Williams did not examine Gregory thoroughly. Amongst other things, Dr Williams should have examined the calves, and noted his findings. He should have included DVT and pulmonary embolism as a differential diagnosis to explain the clinical features, even if this was not his working diagnosis.

The medical records of the clinical examinations followed an identical structure. It was likely that Dr Williams merely selected preformatted text on his computer when constructing his notes. Bronchodilators were prescribed, without evidence of bronchospasm, even though bronchodilators had probably not been of benefit previously.

Gregory was a fit man who had run half-marathons; he suddenly "needed" recurrent use of bronchodilators and antibiotics.

The radiologist reporting the first chest x-ray soon after the holiday suggested a CT scan. By the time Dr Williams considered further investigation after the second chest x-ray, Gregory was dead.

Although a simple CT scan without contrast was not the correct investigation at that time, it is likely that if Dr Williams had discussed with the radiologist the clinical problem, together they would have recognised that pulmonary embolism was likely. Then they would have concluded that inpatient investigation, with close monitoring, was mandated.

Even at the time of the second x-ray, three days before Gregory's death, there was still time for discussion between Dr Williams and the radiologist. In addition to any conversation initiated by Dr Williams, it would have been appropriate for the radiologist to contact Dr Williams, particularly after the second x-ray. It is tragic that Dr Williams proceeded in isolation and did not consult with others.

What is the obligation of practitioners to communicate with one another? The Royal Australian College of General Practitioners' definition of the role of the general practitioner includes "comprehensive care". The same applies to the American and European Colleges. Dr Williams did not understand what the problem was and he did not deliver comprehensive care. If he had consulted with a colleague (general practitioner or radiologist) he would likely have made the correct diagnosis, and Gregory would have survived.

Clinical Principles

It is axiomatic that coughing blood following air travel means a pulmonary embolus until proven otherwise. It is difficult to comprehend that Dr Williams did not understand this.

The risk of pulmonary embolism after air travel is also well understood by the nonmedical community. Prevention of DVT is one of the reasons that air travellers are advised to exercise their legs frequently during long flights.

Gregory needed a D-dimer assay and/or a ventilation perfusion lung scan and/or a CT pulmonary angiogram. If any of these had been arranged, Gregory would likely have received appropriate therapy and would not have died.

ASTHMA DURING PREGNANCY

History

Sharon Monty was 21 years old and 30 weeks pregnant when she presented to a small rural hospital at 19:00 h very short of breath. She had a long history of asthma. The hospital records showed an oxygen saturation of 98%, a pulse rate of 132 bpm, respiratory rate of 20/min, blood pressure of 120/80 mmHg and a temperature of 37°C. There was no detail in the notes of her ability to speak in full sentences or of her use of accessory respiratory muscles.

When the on-call medical officer, Dr Fleur Jackson, was contacted she did not attend the hospital, rather she prescribed salbutamol via a nebuliser, and instructed that Sharon be sent home after her breathing had improved. Sharon could return to the hospital if she became uncomfortable again. After the salbutamol, Sharon's breathing improved and she was allowed home.

It was midnight when Sharon returned to the hospital, very dyspnoeic and more severely unwell than she had been earlier in the evening. On this occasion the oxygen saturation was 93%, pulse rate 136 bpm and respiratory rate 36/min. Sharon was admitted to the hospital on the telephone advice of Dr Jackson, who again did not attend. Dr Jackson suggested repeated doses of salbutamol and oxygen. She stated that she would visit Sharon in the morning prior to commencing her consulting session.

At midday when Dr Jackson eventually arrived at the hospital to visit Sharon it was 17 hours following Sharon's first presentation the previous evening. By now Sharon was exhausted. She was using her accessory muscles of respiration and could hardly speak. Her oxygen saturation was 88% with a pulse rate of 140 bpm, a respiratory rate of 26/min and systolic blood pressure of 76 mmHg. A prominent bilateral wheeze was present, more particularly noted at both bases. Dr Jackson contacted the base hospital who advised steroids and urgent transfer.

On arrival at the base hospital Sharon was placed in an induced coma where she remained. Sharon had a pneumothorax, confirmed on x-ray. Two weeks following arrival at the base hospital Sharon's twins, who had died in utero, were delivered. The following week Sharon required a laparotomy to drain an abscess. Three weeks later Sharon died, with multiorgan failure.

Legal Issues

Sharon's family sued Dr Jackson in negligence for nervous shock and for the loss of domestic services and income under Lord Campbell's Act. They alleged that Dr Jackson had failed to assess Sharon when she first presented to hospital, and again when she returned several hours later. Prompt assessment would have alerted her to the imminent calamity. Sharon would have received earlier, more aggressive therapy. The nursing staff would not have been left unsupported.

Dr Jackson's conduct was not supported by any expert evidence. Respiratory physicians provided conflicting reports about whether Sharon and her twins would have survived with earlier assessment and referral to the base hospital.

The case settled at mediation.

Discussion

Dr Jackson was on-call to manage patients at a rural hospital. Although Sharon was pregnant and clearly unwell when she first presented to hospital, Dr Jackson, for whatever reason, chose not to examine Sharon, and expert care at the base hospital was delayed. Even when Sharon came back to the hospital at midnight more unwell, Dr Jackson deferred her assessment of Sharon for another 12 hours.

Dr Jackson failed to understand that asthma late in pregnancy is more serious than otherwise. The diaphragm is pushed upwards by the gravid uterus and lung capacity is reduced. Patients like Sharon are prone to deteriorate rapidly without proper care.

Dr Jackson did not ask the nurses during either of the telephone calls for details of Sharon's breathing. How laboured was it? Was she using accessory muscles of respiration? These are important questions in a patient with acute asthma, particularly so in one who is pregnant.

There is also the question of the relationship between the doctor and the nursing staff. It is not uncommon for very junior nurses without much clinical experience to be working in rural hospitals. Did Dr Jackson believe that her nurses were capable of managing a pregnant patient with severe asthma? Or did she just hope that Sharon would be better in the morning?

The case highlights the need to be diligent and not to take short-cuts in the assessment and management of patients. In the majority of cases, doctors can get away with taking short-cuts. But medical conditions and patients do not always follow the desired script. Severe illness can occur during the night. It is not always appropriate to wait until the morning. If one repeatedly takes short-cuts in medicine, inevitably they will lead to negative outcomes.

Rural patients are well aware of the difficulties of rural medical practice, and respond well to requests from their doctor to defer appointments if something urgent arises. If Dr Jackson had visited Sharon at midnight and then needed to postpone review of other patients to later in the morning, those other patients would likely have understood, and not begrudged Dr Jackson a few hours of sleep. Sharon and her twins may have survived.

Clinical Principles

Being on call at a rural hospital may be a 24-hour responsibility. This is taxing on the doctor and the doctor's family. It is the lot of the rural practitioner. Most are able to organise their life and to prioritise their workload as required. Review of patients with clearly benign conditions may be deferred, in order to be able to review urgently those with potentially serious ailments. The necessary skill is to correctly and efficiently identify and distinguish between benign and potentially serious situations.

DYSPNOEA

History

Skye Bannister was born in 1987, and was three years old when her father died suddenly, aged 33 years. Skye had an elder brother, Andrew, who was born in 1985. Skye's mother had ischaemic heart disease in her fifties, and remained well on treatment. Prior to his death Mr Bannister was separated from Skye's mother, and had another daughter, Deborah, born in 1989.

Skye was in good health until she was 18 years old. She became acutely unwell in December 2005, with chest pain at rest. She had been taking an oral contraceptive tablet but was not known at the time to have any other risk factor for venous thrombosis or pulmonary embolism. She had no fever or headache. Skye attended the local regional community hospital and was assessed by the general practitioner on duty at the hospital that evening, Dr Bruce Prince.

The blood pressure was normal at 114/70 mmHg and the pulse was rapid at 102/min. There was mild tachypnoea, 18/min (reference 14/min). Skye was afebrile, the oxygen saturation breathing room air was 97% (normal, reference >96%) and the breath sounds were vesicular (normal). Dr Prince noted some tenderness over the left anterior chest. Examination otherwise was unremarkable.

The machine-generated ECG report recorded abnormal right axis deviation and abnormal low QRS voltage in the limb leads. Dr Prince noted the absence of ST-T wave changes on the ECG, and ignored the abnormalities highlighted on the machine-generated report.

Although Skye did not have malaise, fever, abdominal pain or headache, Dr Prince diagnosed pleurodynia (lancinating chest pain or abdominal pain, associated with fever, malaise and headache, often with Coxsackie B viral infection). Dr Prince prescribed paracetamol. He did not request lung scanning or specialist review.

Over the next few months Skye experienced cough and dyspnoea, and was reviewed by her regular general practitioner, Dr Asif Rahman. She did not have fever, or signs to suggest bacterial infection. Skye's symptoms persisted despite various antibiotics, and she became increasingly short of breath, and generally unwell. After several reviews, Dr Rahman prescribed iron supplements, although there was no evidence of iron deficiency.

Skye remained unwell through the winter of 2006, and developed orthopnoea and wheeze, for which Dr Rahman prescribed salbutamol and prednisone. Skye developed abdominal discomfort, and was ultimately admitted to hospital with hypotension, tachycardia and tachypnoea.

The electrocardiographic changes which had been present the previous year persisted. In addition, there was now voltage evidence of left atrial enlargement. There was elevation of troponin and liver enzymes, consistent with cardiac failure and hepatic congestion.

Although Skye was conscious, the medical and nursing staff at the hospital were unable to record her blood pressure. Dr Rahman was contacted by telephone, and advised rapid infusion of normal saline. A chest x-ray showed cardiomegaly. Skye remained unwell and was oliguric "despite" three litres of fluid intravenously. Later that evening, at the request of her family, Skye was transferred to a city teaching hospital, 45 minutes away by road.

In addition to the previously documented signs, Skye now had a gallop rhythm and pulmonary crepitations. A chest x-ray confirmed cardiomegaly and left ventricular failure, and an echocardiogram showed left ventricular dilation and severe global hypokinesia. The ejection fraction was ~20%. Skye had thrombosis of the left subclavian vein, and pulmonary embolism. Antibodies to cardiolipin were present.

Despite introduction of appropriate medical therapy (including digoxin, carvedilol, frusemide, ramipril, spironolactone, warfarin, aspirin and a short course of prednisone) Skye's cardiac function did not improve. She required a mechanical left ventricular assist device. A biopsy of the left ventricle showed changes of dilated cardiomyopathy. Her course was complicated by atrial flutter, transient cerebral ischaemia and renal impairment.

Skye received a heart transplant in 2008. Her convalescence thereafter was complicated by rejection and stroke. Eight years following cardiac transplantation Skye remained generally unwell. She was unable to drive her car and unable to work because of presyncope and anxiety, although she was free of cardiac failure.

Legal Issues

Skye sued Doctors Prince and Rahman, because failure to diagnose cardiomyopathy sooner than was the case resulted in a worse outcome than would have been the case if the diagnosis of cardiomyopathy had been made earlier.

Genetic testing showed that Skye had a mutation of the phospholamban gene, which likely accounted for her cardiomyopathy. It transpired that her sister Deborah also had cardiomyopathy, and required cardiac transplantation in 2012. At the time of writing, Deborah had not yet been tested for genetic mutations. Her brother Andrew did not have the phospholamban mutation and did not have cardiomyopathy. It is likely that Skye and Deborah inherited from their father a genetic defect that caused cardiomyopathy.

Expert witnesses for the defence and for the plaintiff agreed that cardiomyopathy was present in 2006. The experts agreed that poor R wave progression and low voltage QRS complexes in the limb leads in 2006 were likely associated with cardiomyopathy, and not due to any other pathology. Those changes had been present the previous year.

Defence experts maintained that even if cardiomyopathy had been diagnosed in 2005, treatment would not likely have altered the outcome. Defence witnesses opined that abnormal right axis deviation may have been due to chronic asthma or emphysema, neither of which was the case. The plaintiff's experts considered that abnormal right axis deviation was likely due to recurrent pulmonary embolisation.

The plaintiff's experts considered that earlier treatment of cardiomyopathy would likely have reduced the rate of progression of cardiac failure, and would have allowed any procedures or interventions to have been undertaken before Skye became as unwell as she did.

The case settled at mediation.

Discussion

When Skye presented to the community hospital in December 2005 she probably had systemic venous thrombosis and pulmonary embolism. She was predisposed to venous thrombosis because she had antibodies to cardiolipin (not known at the time) and was using an oral contraceptive tablet. She also had cardiomyopathy, although she was unaware of it at the time. Poor R wave progression and low voltage QRS complexes were likely due to cardiomyopathy, and right axis deviation was likely due to previous pulmonary embolism. Poor R wave progression was not due to anterior myocardial infarction, and low voltage QRS complexes were not due to a pericardial effusion.

Although Skye did not have a history of malaise, fever, abdominal pain or headache, Dr Prince diagnosed pleurodynia. Dr Prince either did not recognise the abnormalities highlighted in the machine-generated ECG report or chose to ignore them and did not suggest specialist review.

Even if pleurodynia had been the correct diagnosis, pleurodynia did not account for any of the ECG abnormalities. Accordingly, Dr Prince should have requested specialist review to determine what pathology did account for the ECG abnormalities. Skye would then have had a chest x-ray and echocardiogram; cardiomyopathy would have been diagnosed sooner than was the case, and treated appropriately; and she was not likely to have become as unwell as she did so quickly.

Skye consulted Dr Rahman on several occasions in 2006. Cough, which was probably due to pulmonary congestion secondary to cardiomyopathy, did not resolve with antibiotics. Skye reported increasing dyspnoea, and ultimately had orthopnoea and wheeze. When Skye became increasingly severely unwell, Dr Rahman arranged hospitalisation, although he still had not considered that Skye had cardiac failure. It was only when staff at the hospital were unable to record Skye's blood pressure, and the family intervened, that specialist review was arranged.

Once Skye was admitted to the teaching hospital she was appropriately treated, by which time cardiomyopathy was advanced and Skye required heart transplantation.

Clinical Principles

When Skye presented to the community hospital with cough, tachycardia and tachypnoea in the context of oral contraceptive use, pulmonary embolism should have been retained amongst differential diagnoses to explain the clinical features until pulmonary embolism was excluded. It is more likely than not that appropriate investigations (including ventilation-perfusion lung scanning and/or CT pulmonary angiography) would have confirmed the presence of pulmonary embolism.

In addition to the probability of pulmonary embolism, Dr Prince should have appreciated that chest pain in men and women of any age may be due to myocardial ischaemia; serial electrocardiograms and measurements of troponin were indicated.

The ECG changes were not due to pleurodynia, and warranted investigation on their own merit. It was not appropriate to ignore the ECG abnormalities, irrespective of whether or not it was thought that the abnormalities were associated with pleurodynia.

Dr Rahman saw Skye on several occasions and prescribed antibiotics, although there was no evidence for bacterial infection. He did not consider that dyspnoea may have been of cardiac origin.

When dyspnoea does not respond to treatment, or recurs, it is important to exclude potentially lethal pathology, and it is never appropriate to presume a benign diagnosis until potentially lethal diagnoses are effectively excluded. This is best achieved by considering various pathologies that may cause dyspnoea (including lung disease, heart disease, pericardial disease, anaemia, sleep apnoea, obesity, hypothyroidism and depression).

Progressive dyspnoea and orthopnoea in the absence of progressive lung disease, anaemia, sleep apnoea, hypothyroidism and depression is due to cardiac failure unless proved otherwise. In this case cardiac failure was not considered until Skye had severe left ventricular dysfunction, which was by then refractory to medical therapy.

PALPITATIONS

History

Lydia Milton first experienced palpitations in 2007 when she was 12 years old. She said that she felt missed beats occasionally, always at rest, and not associated with menstrual periods or other circumstances. Her palpitations became more frequent during Year 11 at high school in 2012. She did not smoke or use alcohol or illicit drugs. She drank little caffeine and did not use bronchodilators. Routine blood tests including thyroid function were normal.

During her final year at high school Lydia experienced fatigue, pelvic pain unrelated to menstruation, nausea and bouts of diarrhoea alternating with constipation. She was prescribed butylscopolamine by her general practitioner and was referred for surgical review. Abdominal examination was normal and the only abnormality on CT scanning was a possible small left ovarian cyst. No abnormality was detected in the gastrointestinal tract at gastroscopy and colonoscopy in August 2013.

The gastroenterologist noted that Lydia had frequent ventricular ectopic beats while she was sedated for the procedures, and during recovery afterwards. Lydia was then referred to Dr Deborah Hume, a cardiologist in the rural city near where she lived.

Dr Hume noted the history of palpitations and the recently documented ventricular ectopic beats. She recorded that Lydia's palpitations may occur a few times in a day, but were never disabling. Lydia said that she had blacked out on three occasions. Once was in 2010 after running approximately 1 km. Before and after that she had been able to run longer distances without any problem. On another occasion Lydia felt light-headed and fainted while welding on a hot day. On a third occasion early in 2013 she had felt cold and nauseous while sitting in a classroom. She walked outside, felt faint and blacked out briefly. She recovered promptly on every occasion and she was not incontinent. She had no seizures. Lydia had no family history of cardiac arrhythmias or sudden death.

Her pulse rate was 50 bpm and her blood pressure was 115/70 mmHg. Physical examination was unremarkable. The electrocardiogram showed mostly sinus rhythm, and some monomorphic ventricular ectopic beats with a left bundle branch block pattern (positive in leads I and aVF and negative in lead V2, suggesting that the ectopic beats arose in the left or right ventricular outflow tract). The ectopic beats were suppressed during exercise to 9 mins 28 secs of the Bruce protocol. Exercise was limited by fatigue at 99% of her predicted maximum heart rate. Lydia had no palpitations, chest pain or inappropriate dyspnoea. There was no ST segment displacement, and the QT interval was normal throughout. An echocardiogram at rest showed normal left ventricular contraction. There was normal augmentation of contraction with exercise. The heart appeared normal at MRI scanning.

Dr Hume discussed management options with Lydia and her family. Although Lydia was not bothered by her ectopic beats, Dr Hume prescribed flecainide 50 mg twice daily to control the ectopy. Lydia's palpitations probably became less frequent, but she felt profoundly unwell on flecainide. Thinking that medical therapy had failed, Dr Hume referred Lydia to Dr Desmond Liu, a cardiac electrophysiologist in a capital city, for an opinion on further treatment.

Dr Liu reviewed Lydia's history and the investigations and treatment by Dr Hume. He noted that Lydia was increasingly unwell since commencing flecainide. Dr Liu suggested an electrophysiological study to locate the origin of the ectopic beats, and radiofrequency ablation if there was a single origin for the ectopics. These procedures were performed in December 2013, after Lydia completed her high school examinations.

Catheters were placed via femoral veins to the right heart. A single catheter was advanced retrogradely via the femoral artery to the ascending aorta, and into the left ventricle. Dr Liu performed the procedure under light sedation, so as not to suppress the ectopic beats. He did not describe any difficulty mapping the summit of the interventricular septum within the aortic root or within the left ventricle, using computer-generated 3D images and fluoroscopy to assist with catheter placement. He said that he encountered no difficulty prolapsing the electrode catheter into the left ventricle.

Detailed mapping revealed unifocal ventricular ectopic beats arising in the right ventricular outflow tract. After application of radiofrequency energy at the right ventricular outflow tract, no ventricular ectopic activity was noted during 30 minutes of observation before withdrawal of the catheters. At the conclusion of the procedure an echocardiogram showed no evidence of haemopericardium, and the ventricles contracted normally. Aortic regurgitation was not noted. Lydia was discharged home the next day.

Lydia commenced rural studies at university the following year, but had to suspend her course because of postural dizziness and exhaustion. She returned to Dr Hume, who again prescribed flecainide, which made Lydia feel worse. She sought a second cardiological opinion in her home city. Lydia now had clinical evidence of severe aortic regurgitation, confirmed on an echocardiogram. Ambulatory monitoring revealed mostly sinus rhythm with only two ventricular ectopic beats during a 24-hour period. As a result of the aortic regurgitation, Lydia was referred for cardiothoracic surgical review. The surgeon recommended surgical evaluation of the valve.

At operation 26 November 2014 there was a linear tear near the edge of the right coronary cusp extending from one end of the leaflet to the other. The aortic valve was otherwise morphologically normal. The leaflet was repaired, with a satisfactory intraoperative result. The tear was thought to be the consequence of perforation of the leaflet during the radiofrequency ablation.

Lydia was initially well, but soon redeveloped severe aortic regurgitation for which she received a bioprosthetic valve replacement on 15 December 2014.

Lydia did not return to university and was advised to avoid activities which may predispose her to infection and endocarditis. She was told that if she had children, it would be best to have them before deterioration of her prosthetic valve. A subsequent valve replacement would likely be required. If she had a mechanical prosthesis, then she would require anticoagulation, which would increase the risk of fetal complications.

Lydia did not return to university and did not resume farm work, hockey or kickboxing which she had enjoyed previously. She worked at a local retailer before marrying and having children.

Legal Issues

Lydia sought compensation for the consequences of radiofrequency ablation, the perforation to the aortic valve leaflet, the repair of the leaflet, the subsequent valve replacement and the risk of adverse events in the future.

Expert witness cardiologists for the plaintiff and for the defence agreed that perforation of the right cusp of the aortic valve occurred during the procedure by Dr Liu on 23 December 2013. Expert witnesses for the plaintiff and for the defence all accepted that radiofrequency ablation was not warranted in the absence of disabling symptoms and in the absence of cardiac dysfunction as a result of ventricular ectopic beats. There was disagreement as to whether such disability was present prior to the ablation.

The major dispute was the cause of the perforation. Expert witnesses for the defence held the view that perforation of the valve leaflet was an unavoidable accident. It was the materialisation of an inherent risk of radiofrequency ablation, a risk that could not be avoided with the exercise of reasonable care. The plaintiff expert witness was prepared to infer from the outcome and the surrounding circumstances of the operation that the perforation must have been due to the application by Dr Liu of inappropriate force against the aortic valve leaflet.

The case is ongoing.

Discussion

The case highlights the need to consider treatment options carefully before proceeding to invasive therapy. Not all conditions are immediately amenable to a quick fix. Many conditions, particularly cardiac conditions, should be managed medically or by observation before proceeding to potentially risky procedures. While impatience may affect a patient's decision-making, medical practitioners need to be more cautious and sometimes counsel against such interventions.

Lydia had experienced occasional missed beats for four years prior to radiofrequency ablation. Ectopic beats were observed to be suppressed during exercise. Lydia had a morphologically normal heart. She had experienced syncope on three occasions, the circumstances of each of which suggested fainting, and did not suggest a malignant ventricular arrhythmia.

Dr Hume prescribed flecainide to suppress the ectopic beats, on the basis of their mere presence, but not on the basis of disabling symptoms and not on the basis of any cardiac dysfunction as a result of the ectopic beats. Flecainide made Lydia feel worse. Dr Liu did not suggest withdrawal of flecainide and a period of observation. Rather, he offered Lydia radiofrequency ablation to suppress or eliminate her ectopic beats.

The consensus was that ventricular ectopic beats required treatment only if symptoms due to the arrhythmia were severe or if it were likely that ventricular dysfunction (if present) was due to a high burden of ventricular ectopy. Lydia may have suffered side-effects from flecainide, but she did not have disabling symptoms from any underlying cardiac abnormality.

Dr Liu utilised 3D mapping to identify the site of origin of ventricular ectopic beats. He mapped not only the right ventricular outflow tract, but also the left ventricular outflow tract in order to be confident of the origin of Lydia's ectopic beats. At some time in the course of the procedure the tip of the electrode catheter on the left side was passed through the right leaflet of the aortic valve, and not between the valve leaflets.

This is a rare but not unknown complication of electrophysiological procedures involving the aorta and left ventricle. It is normal practice to prolapse the curved tip of an electrode catheter between the leaflets of the aortic valve in order to access the left ventricle. To do otherwise is to risk perforation of an aortic valve leaflet. Dr Liu maintained that he prolapsed the electrode catheter through the aortic valve to the left ventricle on one occasion only, without difficulty.

Perforation of the leaflet was not due to thermal injury because radiofrequency energy was applied only at the right ventricular outflow tract (nowhere near the aortic valve leaflet). Accordingly, it must have been the case that the right leaflet of the aortic valve was perforated by inappropriate force being applied to the catheter against the aortic valve leaflet. There had to have been the application of sufficient force via the catheter onto the aortic valve leaflet to perforate the valve. It could not have been damaged in any other way. Gentle prolapsing of the catheter through the valve leaflets would have avoided the injury.

Clinical Principles

Ventricular ectopic beats are common, particularly in women. As a general rule benign ectopic beats which do not cause disabling symptoms, and are suppressed with exercise and are not associated with any structural abnormality of the heart, do not require treatment. In some patients ectopic beats may be aggravated by alcohol, nicotine, caffeine and sympathomimetic drugs (e.g. bronchodilators for asthma). None of these factors applied to Lydia.

Lydia had fainted on three occasions. It was not unreasonable to consider that these episodes may have been caused by a self-terminating ventricular tachyarrhythmia. There was no evidence for this at ambulatory monitoring and no attempt was made at electrophysiological study to induce ventricular tachycardia. Radiofrequency ablation of Lydia's ectopic beats would not prevent fainting, because ectopic beats were not the cause of fainting.

ISCHAEMIC HEART DISEASE

History

Sally Kawolski was first referred to a cardiologist, Dr Ghulam Basri, in 2011 when she was 61 years old. Sally's mother, who had had hypertension and high cholesterol, died aged 69 years following a heart attack. Her father, who had required coronary artery bypass grafting in his 60s, died aged 71 years. Two sisters and two brothers had also required bypass graft surgery. Sally had a history of being overweight, hypertension, hyperlipidaemia and diabetes mellitus.

She also had a previous history of alcohol intemperance, oesophageal varices, gastritis and mild asymptomatic thrombocytopenia ($95–120 \times 10^9$/L, reference $150-450 \times 10^9$/L). Her alcohol intake had been minimal since 2000. Although a liver biopsy in 1991 had shown changes of 'pre-cirrhosis' probably related to alcohol, there was no documented gastrointestinal bleeding at any time, and numerous gastroscopies after 2006 had been normal.

Prior to first seeing Dr Basri, Sally had been referred for a CT coronary angiogram which showed calcific plaque in all three large epicardial arteries. On the CT scan it was considered likely that there was flow-limiting ostial narrowing in the posterior descending branch (PDA) of the right coronary artery (RCA), but not flow-limiting narrowing elsewhere in any of the coronary arteries.

At the time of the CT scan she was 163 cm and 65 kg (body mass index (BMI) of 25 kg/m^2, reference 20–25 kg/m^2, overweight 25–30 kg/m^2, obese >30 kg/m^2). She had been 14 kg heavier (30 kg/m^2) four years previously. Sally had never experienced chest pain, dyspnoea, palpitations or dizziness. Dr Basri noted that Sally's medications included a statin, an angiotensin receptor blocker and oral hypoglycaemic therapy. She had not been prescribed aspirin or beta blockade. Her blood pressure was 150/70 mmHg and the pulse was regular at 70 bpm. Dr Basri requested a selective coronary angiogram. He did not prescribe aspirin or beta blockade.

At coronary angiography there was 25–30% narrowing of the left anterior descending artery (LAD), 50% narrowing in the proximal RCA and 50% narrowing in the PDA (i.e. less narrowing than had been suggested at CT coronary angiography previously). Dr Basri noted that the PDA was small and not suitable for intervention. It was his view that present medications were appropriate, and he did not suggest aspirin or beta blockade. Dr Basri did not suggest an exercise test or other functional assessment of myocardial perfusion.

In March 2012 Sally was on vacation on a cruise ship in Central America when she experienced tight epigastric pain, sweating, nausea and vomiting. She was reviewed promptly by the doctor on board. The electrocardiogram showed evidence of inferior ST elevation myocardial infarction (STEMI), for which she was treated with thrombolytic therapy. Thirty minutes following thrombolysis there was resolution of ST segment elevation indicating that there was restoration of blood flow to the RCA which likely had been obstructed with thrombus when Sally experienced chest pain and ECG evidence of STEMI. She was transferred to hospital at the nearest port for further management.

Although the report of cardiac catheterisation the day following STEMI suggested progressive coronary arterial narrowing in all three coronary arteries, at subsequent comparison with the angiogram performed the previous year there was in fact little change, except for increased narrowing at the origin of the PDA. A ventriculogram acquired during the cardiac catheterisation 24 hours after STEMI revealed localised hypokinesia in the posterobasal segment of the left ventricle, with overall normal ejection fraction. Sally returned to Australia the following week and was reviewed by Dr Basri.

After Sally received thrombolytic therapy, she experienced no further pain and was overall stable. She was now using aspirin, clopidogrel and a beta blocker as well as her other medications. Dr Basri did not suggest any functional assessment, but did advise further coronary angiography and stenting of the PDA. Stenting was performed without any acute complication.

In addition to stenting the PDA, Dr Basri also stented the LAD (at three sites) and circumflex arteries, although there had not been angiographic evidence of flow-limiting narrowing in those vessels, and no stress test had been performed to suggest that revascularisation was required.

After three-vessel coronary artery stenting Sally attended cardiac rehabilitation and her 6-minute walk distance increased from 385 m to 435 m. An echocardiogram showed resolution of the posterobasal hypokinesia.

Legal Issues

Sally sought compensation for myocardial infarction, hospitalisation in Central America and other costs associated with her aborted holiday.

An expert witness cardiologist for the plaintiff argued that aspirin was indicated to reduce the risk of coronary thrombosis because Sally had ischaemic heart disease. There had been no gastrointestinal bleeding or abnormality at gastroscopies after 2006. The expert considered that Sally had proven atherosclerotic coronary arterial disease for which secondary prevention with aspirin was indicated.

An expert witness cardiologist for the defence argued that aspirin was contraindicated because Sally had had mild asymptomatic thrombocytopenia in the past, and had a history of oesophageal varices 20 years previously. Another expert witness cardiologist for the defence argued that aspirin was not indicated for primary prevention of cardiovascular events in diabetic patients.

Neither expert dealt with the fact that Sally had never had any episode of gastrointestinal bleeding, and yet had proven coronary atherosclerosis.

The case settled in 2016 before trial.

DISCUSSION

This case highlights the correct treatment of ischaemic heart disease.

In 2011 Sally had numerous risk factors for ischaemic heart disease. Both parents and four siblings had ischaemic heart disease, and Sally had a history of being overweight, hypertension, hyperlipidaemia and diabetes mellitus. A CT coronary angiogram demonstrated calcific plaque in all three epicardial arteries. Selective coronary angiography revealed no flow-limiting disease for which revascularisation might be considered.

Sally's medications in 2011 included a statin, an angiotensin receptor blocker and oral hypoglycaemic therapy, but did not include aspirin or a beta blocker. She had a remote history of oesophageal varices probably associated with liver disease caused by alcohol, and asymptomatic mild thrombocytopenia. When she stopped drinking alcohol her varices resolved, and gastroscopies after 2005 were normal. Sally had no history of gastrointestinal bleeding at any time. The primary issue in this case was whether Sally should have been prescribed aspirin in 2011, and whether prescription of aspirin would have altered her outcome.

It was the widely held view of cardiologists in 2011 that medical therapy for ischaemic heart disease should include aspirin (to reduce the risk of coronary thrombosis) and statin therapy (to reduce the risk of atherosclerotic plaque rupture and coronary thrombosis, and to reduce hepatic synthesis of atherogenic cholesterol), and angiotensin converting enzyme inhibition (as required and as tolerated for blood pressure control). Beta blockade could be indicated for symptomatic myocardial ischaemia.

In the absence of a compelling bleeding contraindication to aspirin, there was no reason to withhold aspirin. This was because the preventable coronary thrombotic risk without aspirin therapy exceeded the haemorrhagic risk with aspirin therapy. It was ultimately accepted by the defence team that Sally should have been prescribed aspirin in 2011, and that aspirin likely would have reduced the risk of coronary thrombosis in 2012.

The other issue to consider is whether three-vessel stenting was indicated. As a general principle, coronary artery stenting does not improve prognosis in individuals without symptomatic myocardial ischaemia or in patients with predictable angina pectoris at a moderate or high level of work. Prior to acute thrombotic occlusion of the PDA, Sally had not experienced symptomatic myocardial ischaemia. In 2011 there was no angiographic evidence of flow-limiting stenosis in any coronary artery. Stenting was contraindicated.

In 2011, Dr Basri concluded correctly that stenting was contraindicated, but neglected to prescribe aspirin which was indicated. In 2012 Dr Basri correctly concluded that apart from incremental ostial narrowing in the PDA (associated with plaque rupture and healing thereafter) there was no other flow-limiting stenosis in any coronary artery. In the absence of demonstration of symptomatic reversible ischaemia in the myocardium subtended by the PDA, there was no reason to consider stenting.

Following successful thrombolysis in 2012 it was appropriate for Sally to perform an exercise stress test. If Sally had been able to exercise to a moderate level of work without evidence of ischaemia (i.e. absence of chest pain and/or dyspnoea and absence of pathological inferior ST segment depression) then medical therapy alone was indicated.

If at stress testing Sally experienced chest pain and/or dyspnoea, associated with pathological inferior ST segment depression at a low level of work, then it would have been appropriate to discuss with her the potential risks and benefits of stenting the PDA. There would have been no survival benefit from stenting, and there may have been complications including early and late stent thrombosis, and restenosis. Stenting one branch of one artery in a diabetic patient such as Sally may not relieve myocardial ischaemia, particularly in the presence of diabetic small vessel disease. There was no place to consider ‘prophylactic’ stenting of any other vessel in which there was not flow-limiting stenosis.

Although there may not have been any acute complication of stenting, Sally is now at risk of instent restenosis in all three coronary arteries; such risk would have been avoided if stenting had not been performed.

Although it was actually not pertinent for Sally, in diabetic patients with flow-limiting three-vessel coronary artery disease, the risks and benefits of multivessel stenting versus coronary artery bypass graft surgery should be canvassed with the patient. It is often the case in diabetic patients with multivessel disease that surgery provides more durable relief of ischaemia than stenting. Management options may also be considered at a heart team meeting including interventional cardiologists, cardiac surgeons, cardiac anaesthetists and intensivists.

Clinical Principles

In patients with proven atherosclerotic coronary arterial disease (i.e. ischaemic heart disease) medical therapy is always indicated, including aspirin, statin therapy and angiotensin converting enzyme inhibition and beta blockade as required and as tolerated.

In patients with a history of upper gastrointestinal bleeding, proton pump inhibition may be required, and adequate antagonism of platelet aggregation may be achieved with aspirin twice or thrice weekly rather than daily; or clopidogrel, prasugrel or ticagrelor at full or reduced dose. Rarely, antiplatelet therapy must be avoided altogether because of bleeding risk.

Coronary artery stenting has no place in the management of asymptomatic stable ischaemic heart disease. The risks and benefits of stenting must be discussed in patients with predictable myocardial ischaemia.

CHEST PAIN

History

Krystyna Horvat migrated from Europe to Australia in 1997, aged 26 years, and was self-employed as a wedding decorator. She had a family history of ischaemic heart disease and diabetes mellitus, and a personal history of cigarette smoking, obesity, hypertension and hypercholesterolaemia.

In 2002 Krystyna attended the local hospital emergency department because of pleuritic chest pain radiating to her jaw, neck and left arm. She was reviewed promptly by the medical officer who noted the family and personal histories of risk factors. Cardiovascular examination was unremarkable. Serial ECGs two hours apart showed sinus arrhythmia with normal ST segments and normal T waves, and absence of features to suggest acute myocardial ischaemia, pulmonary embolism or pericarditis. The final diagnosis was "pleurisy".

Krystyna first consulted Dr Harriette Jennings (cardiologist) in 2007 because of exertional dyspnoea and chest discomfort. Dr Jennings noted the family and personal history, including the history of possible pleurisy five years previously. A stress echocardiogram was reported as negative for ischaemia at 9 mins 07 secs of the Bruce protocol. Dr Jennings prescribed rosuvastatin, and advised Krystyna to abstain from cigarette smoking and to lose weight.

Dr Jennings wrote, "I am happy to report that the stress echocardiogram was convincingly normal (as I had expected, but good from a reassurance point of view)."

In 2010 Krystyna was referred back to Dr Jennings because of palpitations due to ectopic beats. On the ECG there was T wave inversion in leads V4 and V5, which had not been present previously. A progress stress echocardiogram was reported as negative for ischaemia. Following the second stress echocardiogram Dr Jennings noted that the T wave changes had now resolved. She concluded that the dynamic T wave inversion may have been due to transient pericarditis, although there had been no pleuritic chest pain, no pericardial rub and no ST segment elevation.

Dr Jennings again suggested statin therapy, as well as angiotensin receptor blockade. Aspirin was not prescribed, and nil follow-up was planned. Later in 2010 Krystyna experienced throat pain and consulted her general practitioner who requested a thyroid ultrasound. This revealed a multinodular goitre without tracheal obstruction. A chest x-ray was unremarkable. Throat pain was not explained by the presence of the goitre.

Krystyna was hospitalised in December 2010 for ovarian cystectomy. There was T wave flattening in leads I, aVL and V4–6, and ST-T wave changes in leads II, III, aVF and V3, which had not been present at the same hospital in 2002. The machine-generated report was "Normal ECG".

Two weeks following ovarian cystectomy, and again the following month, Krystyna was reviewed by general practitioners because of lethargy. Iron supplements were prescribed (although there was no evidence of iron deficiency), and an ECG was requested. The ECG was reported, "Sinus rhythm. Nonspecific ST-T wave changes." It does not appear that this result was followed up at the time.

In June 2013, Krystyna presented to her general practitioner because of fatigue and arm weakness for one week. An ECG at the time was reported, "Sinus rhythm 60 bpm. Inferolateral ST-T changes. Possible ischaemia." The appearances on this ECG were different from previous electrocardiograms. On this occasion there was T wave inversion in leads V3–5, which had not been present previously. There was T wave flattening in leads I, II and aVL, and there were ST-T wave changes in leads II, III, aVF and V6. The general practitioner recalled Krystyna and referred her back to Dr Jennings.

At a stress echocardiogram there was approximately 2 mm inferolateral ST segment depression in leads II, III, aVF and V4–6. These findings were not reported until the following year. In her letter to the general practitioner one year after this stress echocardiogram, Dr Jennings wrote, "The baseline echocardiogram was normal, and at post-exercise there was an appropriate increase in left ventricular contractility with a commensurate reduction in left ventricular cavity size. Interestingly, in the late recovery period, about five minutes after the test was ceased, the T waves became inverted in the anterolateral leads."

Dr Jennings reported this as "a negative stress echocardiogram". To explain this view, she wrote, "One must be wary about interpreting an ECG too much with exercise when the baseline ECG is abnormal, but in view of her past history, I wondered if again the ECG changes were a reflection of pericarditis, which can certainly be a recurrent phenomenon." Yet, at no time had Dr Jennings recorded any clinical feature to suggest pericarditis.

The baseline ECG likely was abnormal because of previous myocardial ischaemia and subendocardial infarction. The dynamic ECG changes during recovery were likely associated with ischaemia. It is not known whether the inferior segments of the left ventricle were well visualised on the echocardiogram at peak exercise, and whether inferior wall hypokinesia may have been missed. The observations on this stress echocardiogram (resting ECG changes which had not been present previously, and dynamic ECG changes during recovery) supported a diagnosis of myocardial ischaemia, and did not contradict the family and personal history which indicated an increased risk for ischaemic heart disease.

In September 2014 Krystyna presented to her general practitioner because of neck pain and dyspnoea. There was nil redness or warmth over the thyroid gland. The general practitioner recorded the diagnosis as "thyroiditis", prescribed a nonsteroidal antiinflammatory agent, and wrote a medical certificate for three days. Later that afternoon Krystyna collapsed at home, and died.

At autopsy there was ~80% atherosclerotic narrowing of right coronary artery, and diffuse disease in the other coronary arteries. The thyroid gland appeared normal and there was not evidence of pulmonary aspiration. The cause of death was ischaemic heart disease.

Legal Issues

Krystyna's family sued Dr Jennings for failure to diagnose ischaemic heart disease and failure to manage ischaemic heart disease appropriately, resulting in Krystyna's premature death. The case settled in 2019, without proceeding to trial.

Discussion

Krystyna had a family history of ischaemic heart disease and diabetes mellitus and a personal history of cigarette smoking, obesity, hypertension and hypercholesterolaemia. These factors indicated an increased risk for atherosclerotic ischaemic heart disease. When she attended hospital with chest pain, aged 31 years in 2002, there was no evidence of acute myocardial ischaemia or myocardial infarction. Although the diagnosis at the time was pleurisy, it is impossible to know now whether some or all of the pain experienced by Krystyna in 2002 prior to her hospital attendance was due to transient coronary thrombosis and myocardial ischaemia.

Krystyna experienced exertional dyspnoea and chest discomfort in 2007, at 36 years of age. It would have been appropriate at this time to transfer her immediately by ambulance to the hospital for management of suspected myocardial ischaemia. In the event, she was referred to Dr Jennings for outpatient review.

It was the widely held view amongst cardiologists in 2007, and subsequently, that exertional chest discomfort in the context of a family history of heart disease and diabetes mellitus, and a personal history of cigarette smoking, hypercholesterolaemia, hypertension and obesity, indicated a high likelihood of underlying atherosclerosis (irrespective of the result of a stress echocardiogram).

It was also widely understood in 2007 and thereafter that symptoms due to myocardial ischaemia reported by women were commonly less specific than those commonly reported by men. Accordingly, the index of suspicion for atherosclerotic ischaemic heart disease should be increased when women present with any symptom to suggest myocardial ischaemia.

The language used by Dr Jennings indicated that it is likely she was influenced by confirmation bias. "I am happy to report that the stress echocardiogram was convincingly normal (as I had expected, but good from a reassurance point of view)." Dr Jennings may have been reassured by the likely absence of flow-limiting coronary arterial obstruction; she should not have been reassured as to the absence of coronary atherosclerosis.

It was inappropriate to reassure Krystyna that she did not have ischaemic heart disease on the basis of a negative stress echocardiogram. Rather, it was important to emphasise the need to minimise the risk of myocardial ischaemia, not only with lifestyle measures, but also with appropriate medical therapy.

It was not correct to conclude that the stress echocardiograms excluded ischaemic heart disease. Although the 2007 study suggested the absence of reversible myocardial ischaemia (provided that normal augmentation of contraction of the inferior segments of the left ventricle was seen at peak exercise) at the time of the study, the study did not contradict all the clinical features which made ischaemic heart disease likely. In 2013, the history of fatigue and arm weakness, the new ECG changes before exercise and the dynamic ECG changes during recovery all made myocardial ischaemia very likely.

This case illustrates a commonly encountered flaw in diagnostic practice. Once a diagnosis of ischaemic heart disease has been falsely "excluded" by a negative exercise test on one occasion, it is common to falsely "exclude" the diagnosis thereafter, even in the face of accumulating features to suggest the diagnosis. Dynamic ST-T wave changes were likely due to myocardial ischaemia or subendocardial infarction, and were not due to pericarditis. Further, exertional chest discomfort is commonly due to myocardial ischaemia, and is not commonly due to pericarditis.

Krystyna was unwell with lethargy two weeks after ovarian cystectomy in 2010. An ECG was reported "Sinus rhythm. Nonspecific ST-T wave changes". These new ST-T wave changes were not "nonspecific". Rather, taken in the context of family and personal histories of risk factors for ischaemic heart disease and symptoms consistent with myocardial ischaemia, the ST-T wave changes were "specifically" associated with myocardial ischaemia following ovarian surgery. Unfortunately, it is likely that this ECG was not followed up.

If the ECG changes had been recognised in 2010, then it is likely that diagnostic coronary angiography would have been performed. This would have demonstrated coronary artery disease for which revascularisation was indicated, in addition to medical therapy. Krystyna would likely have been treated appropriately, and would not have died when she did.

In 2013 Krystyna reported fatigue, and weakness in both arms, and an electrocardiogram suggested myocardial ischaemia. The new electrocardiographic changes confirmed ischaemic heart disease. When Krystyna was reviewed by Dr Jennings in 2013, she noted the new changes on the resting electrocardiogram, and noted exaggeration of ECG changes with exercise but concluded that the changes were due to pericarditis, even in the absence of recent pleuritic chest pain and in the absence of ST segment elevation to suggest pericarditis.

Neck pain in 2014 was attributed to thyroiditis, even though there was nil evidence to support this diagnosis. Krystyna died of myocardial ischaemia. At autopsy there was evidence of diffuse coronary arterial disease and there was not evidence of any other cause for death.

It is most likely that Krystyna experienced sudden collapse due to cardiac arrest in ventricular fibrillation, secondary to acute myocardial ischaemia as a result of thrombotic occlusion of the right coronary artery. It is probable that if Krystyna had been treated with appropriate medications for ischaemic heart disease (including aspirin), the risk of sudden death would have been eliminated, or reduced to the extent that it would be more likely than not sudden death would have been avoided.

Clinical Principles

This case is an example of a clinical situation where the probability of ischaemic heart disease was high. The absence of evidence of myocardial ischaemia at an exercise test was most likely assumed to indicate the absence of ischaemic heart disease, and medical therapy for ischaemic heart disease was consequently inadequate.

If Krystyna had been advised that a negative exercise test did not exclude ischaemic heart disease, then she would likely have recognised symptoms (including arm weakness and throat pain) as due to coronary artery disease. In turn the general practitioners would have had a higher index of suspicion for ischaemic heart disease, and would have requested immediate ambulance transfer to hospital when Krystyna presented with symptoms consistent with an acute coronary syndrome.

It is always appropriate to retain potentially lethal diagnoses amongst differential diagnoses to explain a clinical presentation, until those lethal diagnoses are excluded. In this case, underlying atherosclerotic ischaemic heart disease was not excluded by exercise testing.

Whenever possible it is appropriate to compare a present ECG with previous recordings, even if the machine-generated report indicates that the present recording is within normal limits. This is particularly important in a patient with risk factors for ischaemic heart disease, or symptoms to suggest myocardial ischaemia. In this case changes in electrogram morphology over time were most likely due to ischaemia or subendocardial infarction, even though each ECG taken in isolation may have been technically within normal limits.

TOO MANY COOKS

History

Matthew Vella was 51 years old when he experienced palpitations in April 2012. He took himself to the local regional hospital where the staff noted his history of being overweight (~100 kg), obstructive sleep apnoea and hypercholesterolaemia. Up until this time he had been able to work without difficulty as a labourer. At the hospital, electrocardiographic monitoring revealed paroxysmal AF. There was no evidence of myocardial infarction or cardiac failure. Although there were several cardiologists in his home city, he was transferred to a capital city referral hospital for further investigation.

An echocardiogram was reported by a cardiologist. Left ventricular size was at the upper limit of normal, with overall normal or near normal contraction. The left atrium was mildly dilated. No mention was made of the degree of mobility of the interatrial septum or presence or absence of an atrial septal defect. A stress echocardiogram was supervised by a second cardiologist. Matthew reached 104% of his predicted maximum heart rate at 9 mins 21 secs of the Bruce protocol, and stopped because of fatigue. There were frequent atrial and ventricular ectopic beats during exercise. Augmentation of left ventricular contraction with exercise was normal or near normal. There were nonspecific ST-T wave changes on the electrocardiogram at peak exercise. At subsequent ambulatory monitory there was AF during 8 of 24 hours. The ventricular rates during AF were 70–90 bpm.

Matthew was advised to lose weight. He was treated for sleep apnoea and was commenced on a low dose of a beta blocker.

He then remained well until October 2012 when he began to experience exertional chest discomfort. He was readmitted to the same hospital he had been to earlier in the year and was assessed by a third cardiologist. On this occasion he reached 71% of his predicted maximum heart rate at 5 mins 39 secs of the Bruce protocol, and stopped because of chest pain associated with >1 mm inferolateral ST segment depression, and ST elevation in lead aVR. At diagnostic coronary angiography there was approximately 50% narrowing of the left main coronary artery and approximately 90% ostial narrowing of the left anterior descending artery (LAD). There were minor irregularities elsewhere.

The third cardiologist discussed revascularisation options with Matthew who decided on coronary artery bypass grafting the following month. He received three separate grafts: left internal mammary artery (LIMA) to LAD, right internal mammary artery (RIMA) to the intermediate artery (INT) and left radial artery (LRA) to the posterolateral circumflex artery (PLCX). An atrial septal defect, which was noted at intraoperative transoesophageal echocardiography, was closed with a patch. AF did not recur after closure of the atrial septal defect and treatment for sleep apnoea. Matthew's convalescence was uncomplicated and he returned to work 3 months later on light duties.

During 2015 Matthew was sometimes aware of extra beats and missed beats at rest, and sometimes had dull chest discomfort at the onset of exercise. In November 2015, he was assessed by a fourth cardiologist in his home city. An echocardiogram showed normal left ventricular size with normal or near normal contraction. The left atrium was mildly dilated. At ambulatory monitoring there was sinus rhythm with occasional atrial and ventricular ectopic beats. There was no AF.

In December 2015 Matthew presented to the local regional hospital with left shoulder, neck and chest discomfort which had commenced on waking, three hours before he arrived at the hospital. Matthew's discomfort was worse when lying down and was relieved when sitting up. The doctor in the emergency department observed reproducible tenderness on the left side of the neck. The tenderness was aggravated by neck movement. The doctor noted that Matthew worked as a labourer which entailed lifting and carrying weights >10 kg, and that he was able to walk several kilometres without difficulty. There was no electrocardiographic evidence of myocardial ischaemia or pericarditis. There was not elevation of troponin, and the D-dimer test was negative. Thus, Matthew's presentation was not likely due to myocardial ischaemia or pulmonary embolism, and was more likely due of musculoskeletal origin.

Nevertheless, since Matthew had presented with chest pain, and had a history of surgical coronary revascularisation, an exercise stress test was requested. He reached 80% of his predicted maximum heart rate at 9 mins 02 secs of the Bruce protocol without chest pain. There was ~1 mm upsloping ST depression in leads V1 and V2. The junior house officer who had supervised the exercise test discussed the result with the on-call cardiologist, the fifth cardiologist so far involved in Matthew's care. The on-call cardiologist requested coronary angiography, to be performed by Dr Vyan Reddy, the sixth cardiologist to be involved in Matthew's care.

Selective coronary angiography was performed via the right femoral artery. At no stage during this procedure was heparin administered. The left coronary artery was imaged in three views, each of which demonstrated ostial occlusion of the LAD. There was approximately 50% narrowing of the left main coronary artery, as previously, and there was brisk flow to the INT and two posterolateral branches of the circumflex artery. These findings suggested that the LIMA graft to the LAD was patent, and that the native LAD was occluded because of competitive flow via the graft. It was not likely that grafts to the INT or PLCX were patent given that there was brisk flow down the native vessels.

The right coronary artery was imaged in two views, both of which showed only minor irregularities, as previously. Dr Reddy then selectively engaged the LRA graft to the PLCX. As anticipated this graft was poorly opacified and appeared diffusely diseased. Dr Reddy next opacified the right subclavian artery at the origin of the RIMA. As anticipated, there was no flow down the RIMA to the INT. Dr Reddy and a cardiology trainee then attempted on twelve further occasions to selectively engage the diffusely diseased RIMA.

Finally, the LIMA was imaged in two views. As anticipated the LIMA was widely patent.

Matthew recalled that Dr Reddy and the trainee had experienced difficulty obtaining images of the coronary artery grafts. He was under the impression that the trainee was more aggressive than Dr Reddy had been. Towards the end of the procedure Matthew became acutely unwell and felt dizzy. He was transferred to the x-ray department where a CT cerebral angiogram revealed thrombus in the basilar artery.

Matthew was then transferred to the intensive care unit for thrombolytic therapy. He received 90 mg of alteplase (standard dose 0.9 mg/kg) 126 minutes after acquisition of the final image at cardiac catheterisation. He was then transferred to a different capital city referral hospital from the one he had been referred to initially when he had AF, for clot retrieval if required. In the event progress scanning revealed the absence of persistent thrombus and no further vascular intervention was indicated.

An MRI scan showed multiple areas of infarction involving the basal ganglia bilaterally, the right occipital and temporal lobes, the right cerebellar hemisphere, temporal and frontal lobes and the right cerebellar hemisphere. Matthew received in-hospital rehabilitation for two months before he was discharged home. He now has persistent cognitive impairment, impaired judgment, poor insight and impaired vision. He will never be able to return to work.

Legal Issue

Matthew sought compensation for the stroke which occurred during cardiac catheterisation.

His case was supported by the opinion of a cardiologist. The cardiologist considered that the stroke occurred because of the actions and inactions of Dr Reddy. The relevant actions were unnecessary instrumentation of the right subclavian artery, presumably in order to obtain selective engagement of the RIMA, despite the angiographic evidence he had already acquired which showed that the RIMA was either diffusely diseased or occluded. Persistent recurrent attempts to engage the RIMA only increased the risk of stroke, and could not have provided additional useful information that would have influenced subsequent management. The relevant inaction of Dr Reddy was not to administer heparin before or during the catheterisation procedure. This failure could only have increased the risk of thromboembolism.

The case is ongoing.

Discussion

Although the legal claim was against Dr Reddy, the final cardiologist in the chain, the case is largely about the importance of continuity of care and the admonition against too many cooks.

During a period of three years Matthew encountered six different cardiologists, each of whom addressed different aspects of his management. When he had exertional chest pain in October 2012 an exercise test suggested flow-limiting myocardial ischaemia at a low workload. At selected coronary angiography there was ~50% narrowing of the left main coronary artery and ~90% ostial narrowing of the LAD. This was appropriately managed with coronary artery bypass grafting. The atrial septal defect was appropriately closed during the same operation.

As it turned out, only the LIMA graft to the LAD remained patent three years later. The other grafts failed because there was brisk anterograde flow via the native vessels to which the other grafts were applied. In November 2015 Matthew was aware of extra and missed heart beats at rest, and had dull central chest pain at the onset of exercise. He was assessed by a fourth cardiologist. At ambulatory monitoring there were atrial and ventricular ectopic beats, which probably accounted for Matthew's symptoms at rest.

The following month Matthew had left shoulder, neck and chest pain when lying down. This discomfort was relieved when he sat up and there was tenderness in the left neck, worse with movement. The hospital doctor at the time noted that he was able to walk several kilometres without difficulty, notwithstanding the dull central chest discomfort which Matthew had experienced the previous month. At the exercise test Matthew reached a moderately high level of work without chest pain and without electrocardiographic changes to suggest flow-limiting myocardial ischaemia for which redo revascularisation might be required.

Another cardiologist, who had probably never seen Matthew before, and may not have seen him in hospital after the exercise test in December 2015, requested coronary angiography.

Yet another cardiologist, Dr Reddy, became involved thereafter.

Dr Reddy acquired images of the native left and right coronary arteries which showed stable ~50% narrowing of the left main coronary artery. Whereas the LAD had been patent prior to surgery, it was now closed. Since there was brisk anterograde flow via the INT and PLCX, it was likely that the RIMA and LRA grafts were diffusely narrowed or occluded. Nothing was to be gained by proving that as a matter of certainty. Multiple unnecessary attempts to selectively engage the RIMA increased the risk of thromboembolism or embolisation of debris from the aorta to the brain and elsewhere.

Dr Reddy demonstrated diffuse disease in the LRA graft and then turned his attention to the RIMA graft, before imaging the LIMA. He should have done it the other way round. After acquisition of images of the native left and right coronary arteries and the diseased LRA graft, the next relevant vessel to image was the LIMA as it supplied the anterior wall of the left ventricle. If this vessel was patent, then the final vessel image required was the right subclavian artery near the origin of the RIMA. If Dr Reddy had limited the number of attempts to engage the RIMA, Matthew would probably not have had his debilitating stroke.

Clinical Principles

Matthew encountered six cardiologists over three years in his home town, as well as other cardiologists involved in his care at capital city referral centres. It is possible that if a single cardiologist had provided continuity of care over time, clinical decisions may have been different and repeat cardiac catheterisation may have been avoided.

Taken out of context, the presentation in December 2015 with chest pain may have warranted exercise stress testing, even though the history spoke against Matthew's pain being due to myocardial ischaemia. The stress test did not suggest that redo revascularisation was indicated, yet repeat coronary angiography was requested. Would repeat coronary angiography have been arranged if Matthew had a single cardiologist responsible for his care?

There was no excuse for the omission of heparin during cardiac catheterisation. Even if Dr Reddy had delegated to another person the responsibility for administration of heparin, it remained Dr Reddy's responsibility to ensure that heparin was administered.

BREAST LUMPS

This chapter comprises brief stories of five patients.

HISTORIES

Radiologist Suggests Further Investigation

Mary Jones, aged 56 in 1996, attended her general practitioner, Dr Nigel Valentine, for a routine medical review. As part of his assessment Dr Valentine referred Mary for a mammogram. The radiologist was not convinced that the mammogram of the left breast was normal, and recommended further investigations. During the ensuing months Mary returned to Dr Valentine on several occasions for other reasons; he never requested further investigations of Mary's breasts.

In 1997 Mary detected a lump in her left breast and attended a second general practitioner who ordered another mammogram. This mammogram was clearly abnormal; Mary was referred for urgent surgery. She now had a stage two carcinoma, for which she required surgery, radiotherapy and chemotherapy.

Persistent Back Pain

Shiva Khatri, aged 55 in 2000, visited her general practitioner, Dr Leonie Lamble, with recent onset low back pain after lifting a heavy wardrobe. Dr Lamble examined Shiva and ordered an x-ray that demonstrated degenerative changes in the lumbosacral spine. A mammogram the previous year had been normal. Dr Lamble referred Shiva to an orthopaedic surgeon, Dr Boris Mikhailov, who prescribed analgesics and physiotherapy, and requested an MRI scan. Although the radiologist reported suspicious bony changes, Dr Mikhailov was unperturbed and returned Shiva to Dr Lamble for conservative care.

Six months later, when Shiva's pain persisted, Dr Lamble referred Shiva to a second orthopaedic surgeon, who examined her and reviewed the MRI scan. There was marrow replacement in the first sacral segment extending to the left of midline and bridging the cortex.

Shiva had breast cancer with bony metastases.

Initial Imaging Negative

Josephine Martindale, aged 55 in 2001, presented to her general practitioner, Dr Lawrence Carmichael with a lump in her right breast. Dr Carmichael confirmed the presence of a lump, and referred Josephine for a mammogram. Although the appearances were within normal limits, the radiologist suggested an ultrasound. The ultrasound appearances were also within normal limits.

Josephine presented twice more during the next three months, concerned about her breast lump. Dr Carmichael reassured her on each occasion. Five months after her original presentation Josephine visited a gynaecologist who suggested a fine needle biopsy of her breast lump. Dr Carmichael waited another two months (and four further consultations) before referring Josephine to a surgeon for a breast biopsy. The fine needle biopsy was positive and four of 24 nodes in the axilla were positive for carcinoma.

Initial Imaging Suspicious

Linda Forrest, aged 49 in 2003, presented to her general practitioner, Dr Mimi Gonzales, three months after discovering a lump in her left breast. The subsequent mammogram revealed thickening within the left breast and the ultrasound demonstrated architectural distortion within the upper half of the left breast. Dr Gonzales reassured Linda that there was no cause for concern, and suggested review in another year. Ultrasound-guided biopsy the next year revealed an adenocarcinoma for which Linda required a radical mastectomy, radiotherapy and endocrine therapy.

Clinical Diagnosis of Cancer

Miriam Irving, aged 40 in 2011, presented to a general practitioner, Dr Saul Goldblatt, for a routine medical examination. Dr Goldblatt discovered a lump in the right breast and palpable lymph nodes in the right axilla. The clinical diagnosis was breast cancer with spread to lymph nodes. An ultrasound performed the following week was reported as normal. Six months later Miriam saw a different general practitioner who referred her to a surgeon. There was a 6 cm × 8 cm carcinoma in the right breast, with spread to local lymph nodes. Miriam required radical mastectomy.

LEGAL ISSUES

Mary Jones sued Dr Valentine because he had ignored the advice of the radiologist, leading to delayed treatment for breast cancer.

Shiva Khatri sought compensation for delayed care because Dr Mikhailov had reassured Dr Lamble inappropriately that Shiva did not require further investigation.

Josephine Martindale claimed compensation for delayed diagnosis and treatment of breast cancer. She had consulted Dr Carmichael on numerous occasions about her lump. It was only after seeking the advice of a gynaecologist that biopsy was suggested. Even then, Dr Carmichael was tardy in proceeding with investigation.

Linda Forrest also sought compensation for delayed diagnosis and treatment. Dr Gonzales knew there were abnormalities on the mammogram and on the ultrasound, yet she did not seek specialist advice until a year later.

Miriam Irving sued Dr Goldblatt because he did not investigate thoroughly when he found a breast lump and lymphadenopathy.

All these matters settled at mediation.

DISCUSSION

In 1997 the Royal Australian College of General Practitioners and the National Breast Cancer Centre published triple test (clinical examination, mammography and fine needle aspiration cytology) guidelines for the management of breast lumps. The guidelines were based on a 99.6% sensitivity of the triple test to diagnose breast cancer, compared with 85% for clinical examination, 90% for mammography and 91% for fine needle aspiration cytology.

The concept of the triple test may not have been well understood by Dr Valentine in 1996 when Mary Jones first presented. However the triple test was accepted practice thereafter, and should have been implemented in all of these cases.

The Royal Australian and New Zealand College of Radiologists issued an article within the fourth edition of their *Imaging Guidelines* in 2001 about low back pain. The first recommendation was that imaging is required if conservative management of back pain does not resolve symptoms within six to twelve weeks. Shiva Khatri required further imaging much sooner than six months after her presentation.

CLINICAL PRINCIPLES

These cases together illustrate several fundamental principles. The radiologist advised Dr Valentine that further investigation was required. Unfortunately Dr Valentine ignored this advice, to Mary's detriment.

When low back pain persists for several months, further imaging is required to exclude sinister pathology. Although Shiva's back pain may have been initially precipitated by lifting a wardrobe, the ongoing pain mandated further investigation.

Josephine was denied the triple test. Earlier fine needle biopsy likely would have secured the diagnosis of breast cancer and allowed earlier treatment.

Dr Gonzales failed to recognise the significance of the abnormal imaging, and failed to implement the triple test. She could easily have consulted an experienced colleague to discuss further investigation.

Dr Goldblatt denied Miriam the benefit of a biopsy. Miriam's physical signs suggested cancer; cancer should have been retained as the provisional or one of the differential diagnoses until or unless disproved.

A NUMBER OF HEALTH CONCERNS

HISTORY

Jade Byrne was 54 years old in 2015 when she presented to a university hospital with left sided chest pain after running from her car to the office in the rain. At the time she was working full-time as a registered nurse.

She had a family history of coronary artery disease and a personal history of cigarette smoking in the past (~10 pack years), hypercholesterolaemia, hypertension and sleep apnoea. In 2009 she was 170 cm and 120 kg (body mass index (BMI) of 42 kg/m^2, reference 20–25 kg/m^2, obese >30 kg/m^2). Jade also had Hashimoto thyroiditis, asthma, irritable bowel syndrome and a hiatus hernia. Prior to 2015 Jade's medications included thyroid hormone replacement therapy, topiramate and phentermine for weight loss, fluoxetine to antagonise the stimulant effect of phentermine, irbesartan and spironolactone for hypertension, rosuvastatin for hypercholesterolaemia and prednisone for asthma. It was fair to say Jade had a number of health concerns.

When she reached her office an ambulance was called. The officers administered sublingual nitrate spray, with partial relief of pain. Jade's pain subsided further with intravenous fentanyl. At the hospital there were dynamic electrocardiographic changes to suggest transmural inferior ischaemia, but her troponin was not elevated on serial testing.

Jade proceeded to diagnostic cardiac catheterisation by Dr Wang Yong on the day of admission. Images of the left main coronary artery (LMCA) were foreshortened in several views and the origins of the left anterior descending (LAD) and circumflex (LCX) arteries were not well seen. Steep angulated views and magnified views of the LMCA and proximal LAD and LCX were not obtained.

Nevertheless, on the images obtained, after administration of nitroglycerine, there was ~50% narrowing at the origins of the LAD and LCX, and there was post stenotic dilation of the proximal LAD immediately after its origin. There were minor luminal irregularities elsewhere.

Dr Wang commented that the degree of narrowing in the proximal segments of the LAD and LCX may have been less following nitroglycerine than was the case before nitroglycerine. He did not, however, employ intravascular ultrasound or measurement of coronary fractional flow reserve to further assess the narrowings in Jade's arteries.

Notwithstanding Jade's presenting symptoms and proximal narrowing of the LAD and LCX, Dr Wang concluded that the arteries were normal. This wrong conclusion was subsequently accepted by others. Jade continued to experience chest pain in hospital for which she was prescribed isosorbide mononitrate. She was subsequently discharged without any further investigation or treatment.

Jade continued to experience chest pain on exertion throughout 2015. She used sublingual nitrate spray with benefit. She also experienced aching in the left upper arm, relieved with sublingual nitrate spray. She remained a non-smoker.

Although she denied having gastro-oesophageal reflux Jade's endocrinologist said that he believed her pain was due to oesophageal spasm.

In September 2015 Jade presented to the university hospital because of further chest pain. The emergency department intern referred to the previous angiogram report and concluded that Jade's pain was not likely to be of cardiac origin.

Her gastroenterologist believed that Jade may have had two different causes for chest pain: coronary artery spasm and gastro-oesophageal reflux. Although no erosive changes were noted at gastroscopy while on rabeprazole, there was evidence of mild chronic inflammation in the stomach on histologic examination.

Jade continued to see her general practitioner who noted that Jade was having "a lot of angina".

Jade was readmitted to hospital in October 2015 following chest pain, nausea and sweating after walking up stairs. Her pain subsided with rest and sublingual nitrate spray. There was no elevation of troponin.

On this occasion a different emergency department intern concluded that Jade had coronary arterial spasm. A medical registrar noted that Jade had experienced pain on exertion, and sometimes after food. She agreed that Jade may have coronary artery spasm, and requested cardiological review.

Dr Sandra Cole, a cardiology registrar, wrote in the progress notes the following day that Jade complained of chest pain that came only after eating, and not with exercise. Dr Cole accepted the coronary angiogram report that the coronary arteries were normal. She declined to admit Jade under the care of a cardiologist on the basis that Jade had oesophageal spasm. Nevertheless she suggested nifedipine and additional isosorbide mononitrate if others felt that her pain was due to coronary artery spasm.

Jade was later reviewed by the general medical team. Notwithstanding Dr Cole's opinion, the general medical physician retained coronary artery spasm as a differential diagnosis. No further steps were taken and Jade was discharged from hospital.

After discharge, Jade continued to experience chest pain. She reported to her general practitioner persistent chest pain on walking. Her dose of nifedipine was increased and she was referred to a general surgeon. The general surgeon was concerned about the exertional chest pain relieved with sublingual nitrates. Jade was then referred to Dr Ajit Chopra, cardiologist, and to an upper gastrointestinal surgeon. The surgeon arranged an oesophageal motility study, which turned out to be normal. There was no evidence of oesophageal dysmotility.

When Jade saw Dr Chopra, he noted a history of crushing central chest pain on exertion and when bending forward. Although the serum cholesterol had been elevated for several years, and Jade had been treated with rosuvastatin, Dr Chopra thought that she did not have hypercholesterolaemia. He noted that a recent echocardiogram had shown normal left ventricular size and function. Dr Chopra formed the view that Jade had oesophageal spasm and did not review her again after the oesophageal motility study which suggested the absence of oesophageal spasm.

Jade was admitted to a private hospital on 10 December 2015 for laparoscopic gastric bypass and hiatus hernia repair. During the immediate postoperative period Jade experienced severe left chest and left shoulder pain for which she required multiple doses of intravenous fentanyl. No electrocardiogram was performed during the evening, and serum troponin was not measured until the following day.

Jade experienced ongoing chest and shoulder pain, and paraesthesia in the left arm. The first postoperative electrocardiogram was performed at 05:33 h on 11 December 2015. This showed new anterolateral T wave changes. Subsequent electrocardiograms showed evolving anterior myocardial infarction. The initial serum troponin was 294 ng/L (reference <14 ng/L). The serum troponin peaked the following day at 4,581 ng/L. The pattern of rise and fall of troponin indicated myocardial infarction commencing during or soon after surgery.

An echocardiogram in the intensive care unit showed hypokinesia of the apical septum, and adjacent inferior and anterior walls with dilation of the left ventricle and atrium. There was neither apical ballooning nor basal hyperkinesia. The ejection fraction was ~50% (reference >50%).

Dr Chopra was asked to review Jade. He initially interpreted the electrocardiographic and echocardiographic changes as being consistent with takotsubo cardiomyopathy. He subsequently reviewed his opinion and concluded that Jade had had anterior myocardial infarction. He did not advise Jade of his change of opinion.

Jade continued to experience angina pectoris in hospital and her progress echocardiogram showed persistent hypokinesia of the left ventricle, without apical ballooning or basal hyperkinesia.

Based on the report by Dr Wang that the coronary arteries were normal, Dr Chopra thought that Jade had coronary artery spasm. He approved her discharge from hospital.

After Jade was discharged home she complained to her general practitioner that she was not happy with the care offered by Dr Chopra. Jade was referred to another cardiologist who requested an MRI scan of the heart. This showed aneurysmal dilation of the anteroseptal and apical segments of the left ventricle. The left ventricle was dilated overall and the ejection fraction was 32%. The perfusion images suggested ischaemia in the lateral wall of the left ventricle. There was mild mitral regurgitation and there was thrombus at the apex of the left ventricle, for which Jade was anticoagulated with warfarin.

On 04 March 2016 a second coronary angiogram was performed, by Dr Marios Christoforou. Dr Christoforou reported 90% ostial narrowing of the LAD and 30% narrowing at the origin of the LCX. The images of the proximal vessels were foreshortened, as before. Although there was dyskinesia in the myocardium subtended by the left anterior descending artery, and although the MRI scan suggested reversible ischaemia in the territory supplied by the circumflex artery, Dr Christoforou proceeded to stent the LAD, and ballooned the origin of the LCX, but did not place a stent in the LCX.

Following Dr Christoforou's treatment, Jade continued to experience angina pectoris on any more than mild physical exertion.

With medical therapy including nifedipine, sacubitril, spironolactone and valsartan, left ventricular function improved, but remained impaired. An echocardiogram on 21 March 2018 showed persistent left ventricular and left atrial dilation, akinesia of the apex and adjacent segments and mild hypokinesia of the inferoseptal region. There was mild mitral regurgitation and the left ventricular ejection fraction was 45%. At an echocardiogram on 21 September 2018 inferior wall hypokinesia was reported as moderate, and the ejection fraction was 42%. Despite medical therapy Jade experienced fatigue on mild exertion and was unable to resume full-time work.

Legal Issues

Jade sought compensation for the consequences of delayed diagnosis of coronary artery narrowing due to atherosclerosis. Expert witness cardiologists for the defence accepted that Jade experienced exertional chest pain in the context of multiple risk factors for coronary artery disease, but argued that her pain was not typical angina pectoris. They argued that the degrees of narrowing of the LAD and LCX were less than what Dr Wang's angiogram had shown. All of the expert witnesses for the defence accepted that Jade had experienced myocardial infarction during the afternoon of 10 December 2015. One of the experts subsequently argued that Jade had takotsubo cardiomyopathy.

One of the defence experts accepted that Dr Wang's angiogram report was wrong and said that this influenced subsequent assessments. This expert considered that Jade had lost an opportunity for timely treatment of myocardial infarction on 10 December 2015. He speculated that the surgeon would have obstructed management of myocardial infarction by angioplasty because of the risk of bleeding associated with antagonism of platelet aggregation and administration of heparin.

An expert witness for the plaintiff analysed Dr Wang's angiogram and disagreed with Dr Wang's conclusion that the arteries were normal. This witness was also critical of Dr Chopra's preoperative and postoperative assessments. He questioned the rationale for Dr Christoforou's stenting of the LAD and failure to stent the LCX.

The case is ongoing.

Discussion

When Jade presented to hospital in March 2015 with exertional chest pain in the context of all of the risk factors she had for ischaemic heart disease, it was likely that her exertional chest pain was due to myocardial ischaemia. The angiographic images obtained by Dr Wang were inadequate to exclude flow-limiting stenosis at the origins of the LAD and LCX. Even with the images obtained, Dr Wang incorrectly concluded that the coronary arteries were normal. This report inevitably influenced subsequent observers. What might have been a simple problem was converted by this error into a maze of issues centred on Jade's comorbidities.

When Jade presented again to hospital in October 2015 with chest pain after walking up stairs, the emergency department doctors correctly concluded that Jade had myocardial ischaemia. Dr Cole either did not elicit the history of exertional chest pain and response to nitrates, or chose not to record it. Based on the history she recorded, and her acceptance of Dr Wang's angiography report, Dr Cole declined Jade's admission under cardiology. It is likely that if Jade had been admitted under cardiology, her history of exertional chest pain would have been recognised and her initial angiogram would have been reviewed.

Given Jade's ongoing symptoms despite medical therapy, it is probable that further investigation would have been arranged. This could have included repeat coronary angiography with care to acquire optimal views of the LMCA, LAD and LCX, with or without intravascular ultrasound and with or without measurement of fractional flow reserve.

The endocrinologist and the general surgeon both recognised that Jade had angina pectoris. A normal oesophageal motility study made oesophageal spasm unlikely.

Dr Chopra must have been influenced by Dr Wang's report of normal coronary arteries. He concluded that Jade's symptoms were probably due to oesophageal spasm. He did not revise this opinion after the oesophageal motility study. If Dr Chopra had reviewed the initial angiogram in the context of Jade's ongoing symptoms, and if he had accepted the absence of oesophageal dysmotility, he could have revised his opinion and arranged for re-evaluation of Jade's arteries. This would have meant that Jade's coronary artery disease would have been treated optimally before gastrointestinal surgery.

If the doctors and nurses caring for Jade after her gastrointestinal surgery had been aware that Jade had a history of exertional angina pectoris, and had coronary atherosclerosis proven at angiography, they would have immediately considered an acute coronary syndrome when Jade experienced severe chest pain immediately after her surgery. This would have permitted thoughtful consideration by the surgeon, cardiologist, cardiothoracic surgeon, anaesthetist and intensivist about management options. Jade was denied the opportunity to have these options properly considered before there was permanent myocardial damage and functional disability.

Clinical Principles

When a patient with multiple risk factors for coronary artery disease presents with exertional chest pain and dynamic electrocardiographic changes to suggest myocardial ischaemia, the possibility of significant coronary arterial obstruction should be considered until such a diagnosis is adequately excluded. The presence of ostial narrowing of the LAD and LCX, with poststenotic dilation in the LAD, made it likely that Jade had flow-limiting narrowing which was not obvious on the angiographic images obtained. This should have led to further evaluation of the lesions.

Dr Cole's assessment of Jade was flawed in that she failed to appreciate that Jade had presented with exertional chest pain. She failed to critically examine the evidence on which a diagnosis of normal coronary arteries was made. These failures likely delayed Jade's correct diagnosis.

Dr Chopra failed to complete his preoperative assessment in that he did not review the images on which a diagnosis of normal arteries was made by Dr Wang. Dr Chopra also failed to reconsider the diagnosis of coronary artery disease when the oesophageal motility study was normal.

Any patient who complains of severe chest pain following surgery should be managed for suspected coronary syndrome until such a diagnosis is excluded and replaced with alternative explanations for symptoms. In this case myocardial ischaemia was not suspected until the day after myocardial infarction.

Doctors may inaccurately record or interpret a history. They may from time to time make a wrong diagnosis. When a patient continues to suffer symptoms, prior assessments must be revisited. This is not a matter of second-guessing others, but ensuring that patients are properly evaluated. Perpetuating previous mistakes is not acceptable. Time and again, especially in hospital settings, an initial history is accepted as a given, repeated by every subsequent examiner, and used as the basis for management decisions. Diligence and an open mind may avert this problem.

A SICK INFANT

History

In 2003, Kylie Miller, then aged two years and three months, woke up one night with severe abdominal pain and vomiting. Mrs Miller took Kylie to their usual general practitioner, Dr Bruce Holmes, the following morning. Dr Holmes considered that she might have been suffering from constipation. He did not examine Kylie's abdomen and did not measure her temperature. The management plan was to increase her fluid intake and review if needed.

Over the following two days the abdominal pain continued, and Kylie developed fever and diarrhoea. It is not known if fever was present at the initial consultation, as the temperature was not recorded. At this second consultation Dr Holmes examined Kylie. He noted an elevated temperature and concluded that she was suffering from gastroenteritis. Palpation of the abdomen was distressing for Kylie. He recommended that she take an electrolyte supplement.

Two days later Kylie's mother called an after hours locum, who examined Kylie and considered that she may have been suffering from appendicitis. After the locum left the house, Mrs Miller phoned Dr Holmes to advise him of the opinion of the locum. Dr Holmes laughed at the suggestion, and said that appendicitis did not occur in patients as young as this.

When Kylie had not improved two days later, Mrs Miller called for an ambulance. Kylie was transferred to the local hospital, where she remained in the waiting room for two hours until the doctor was able to see her. Kylie was reluctant to have her abdomen examined, because of the discomfort she had experienced previously. When she was assessed, the provisional diagnosis was appendicitis. She remained in hospital overnight.

At 09:30 h the following morning Kylie was examined by a consultant surgeon who detected severe tenderness in the right lower quadrant, and suggested that she should be transferred to a specialist paediatric hospital. Kylie watched a children's program on television, while waiting for her father to arrive. When Mr Miller arrived one hour later, Kylie seemed somewhat more comfortable than she had been the night before. The decision was then made by the hospital staff that Kylie was less ill than previously thought, that she was probably suffering from gastroenteritis, and that it would be safe for her to return home. The advice of the consultant surgeon was ignored.

Abdominal symptoms continued over the following four days and Kylie developed a high fever. She was examined once more by an evening locum who considered that she was suffering from appendicitis, and referred her to the regional children's hospital where she was examined by a paediatric surgeon. The paediatric surgeon made the correct diagnosis of a ruptured appendix, which was confirmed following an ultrasound scan of the abdomen.

Laparotomy revealed a ruptured appendix and peritonitis. Following appendicectomy and peritoneal lavage, she remained in intensive care for two days, during which time she received intravenous antibiotics, fluids and morphine.

Kylie was then transferred to a general ward, where she remained for a further two weeks. She required intravenous feeding for the first five days, and was left with an 80 mm × 5 mm keloid abdominal scar.

Legal Issues

Kylie's parents sought compensation relating to the delayed diagnosis and treatment of appendicitis. The case was settled at mediation.

Discussion

This case illustrates the difficulty of reaching a firm diagnosis in a young child. Practitioners caring for young children need to develop a high level of clinical skill, and should not become over reliant on investigations.

One must not forget that basic examination and focused observational techniques are of great value in reaching an accurate diagnosis, even though this is a particular problem in young children who may be frightened of the strange environment in a medical clinic. There are also other situations where communications between practitioner and patient are suboptimal, such as language barriers.

Although many different languages are spoken in Australia, it is usually possible to establish means to communicate adequately. A patient may self-select a doctor familiar with their own language, or the patient may be accompanied by an interpreter familiar to the patient. Interpreter services may be available in person or by telephone or via the internet.

Effective communication in some of the remote small Indigenous Australian communities may be particularly difficult. In these places the sole remote area nurse may be the only one who speaks English. One example of ineffective communication was a 13-year-old Indigenous Australian boy who was unable to give to the nurse an accurate history of his sore back. He became paraplegic because of a spinal abscess.

Some of the larger Indigenous Australian communities have retained their original languages, with only a very few having any English. One example is the community of Wadeye in remote Northern Territory where there are around 2,000 Indigenous Australians. The school teachers and health workers have no chance of mastering their different languages of Murrinh-patha, Magati Ke, Marri Ngarr, Murrinh Kura and Marri Tjevin. Health workers need to be sufficiently skilled in communication to manage such patients where there are both minimal language skills and minimal investigative resources.

Kylie's ruptured appendix was confirmed with ultrasound. This investigative tool is not readily available in many circumstances. In some remote areas of Australia there is no service at all. Patients may need to travel 500 km or more for investigation. This may be a critical impediment to care for a patient with an urgent problem.

Kylie presented to a general practitioner or hospital doctor on no fewer than eight occasions before the correct diagnosis was established (although at least two of the doctors suspected the diagnosis). It is of concern that Dr Holmes had no understanding of the possibility of appendicitis in a patient of this age. It would have been an easy matter to turn to a reference source (telephone, online or textbook) to determine whether appendicitis was a possible diagnosis in such a patient.

What is of significant importance is the understanding of a mother that her child is ill. When a child presents on multiple occasions because of the mother's concern, it is an unwise doctor who reaches a benign diagnosis without carefully eliminating potentially serious diagnoses.

Of value in the diagnosis of appendicitis, particularly when ultrasound is not readily available, is the Mantrels score (score one for each of Migration of pain, Anorexia, Nausea/vomiting, Rebound pain, Elevated temperature and Shift of white cell count to the left; score two each for Tenderness in the right lower quadrant and Leucocytosis).

Score <5	appendicitis unlikely
Score 5–6	appendicitis possible
Score 7–8	appendicitis likely
Score is 9–10	appendicitis highly likely

Kylie's score was at least seven (anorexia, vomiting, rebound pain, fever and tenderness; she may also have had a leucocytosis).

Another factor to be considered is the variation of symptoms over time. Kylie appeared less distressed when she was distracted by a program on television some hours after her admission to hospital on the first occasion. This variation of symptoms is not unusual, particularly in young children.

The locum doctor reached the correct diagnosis at an early stage of the illness and his opinion was given no credence. When Kylie was admitted to the regional hospital no one seems to have understood the fluctuating nature of symptoms in a young child. It is difficult to understand why an ultrasound was not performed prior to Kylie being discharged from hospital the first time.

The delay in diagnosis has likely resulted in a larger and more unsightly scar than would have been the case with earlier diagnosis and treatment. It remains to be seen whether Kylie develops adhesions and/or problems with bowel function due to prolonged abdominal sepsis.

Clinical Principles

The most important feature of this case is that a mother usually knows when her young child is ill. It is foolhardy for a doctor not to take this into account.

The more general principle is the need to communicate effectively with the patient or the patient's surrogate. In this case the mother was the surrogate; in other cases the surrogate may be a language interpreter.

On the first occasion Dr Holmes did not examine Kylie. Consequently he did not record his findings, and did not consider potentially serious differential diagnoses. The initial wrong diagnosis probably influenced some of the subsequent incorrect assessments.

AN AVOIDABLE TRAGEDY

HISTORY

Josh Medhurst was seven years of age when he developed abdominal pain, vomiting and a sore throat while on school holidays with his parents, Ed and Julie. Julie did not think Josh was himself. He had not passed a bowel motion for a couple of days. He was quiet and drowsy. She took him to the local medical centre the next day on 10 May 2011, where he was seen by Dr Abdul Saqlain. After a somewhat cursory examination and questioning, Dr Saqlain diagnosed constipation and prescribed a laxative. He told Julie to bring Josh back in for a check-up if he did not improve.

Two days later, on 12 May 2011, Julie returned to the medical centre, where Josh was examined by another general practitioner, Dr Crawford Sampson. By the time of Dr Sampson's examination, Josh had a history of abdominal pain of four days' duration, anorexia, a slight fever and vomiting. Dr Sampson found on examination that Josh had a tachycardia of 100 bpm, a mild pyrexia of 37.8°C, absent bowel sounds and a tender, distended, rigid abdomen. Dr Sampson diagnosed Josh as having acute appendicitis with possible secondary bowel obstruction or rupture of the appendix. He thought Josh was very unwell and called an ambulance to take him to the nearest hospital with a paediatric emergency department. Julie accompanied Josh, while Ed came in later once he received the news.

At about 10:00 h on 12 May 2011, Josh presented to the emergency department at the closest hospital with a paediatric ward. The ambulance officers followed protocol to take Josh to that hospital rather than a tertiary children's hospital. While the hospital had a paediatric ward and some elective paediatric surgery was performed there, it did not have the paediatric surgical services to treat acute conditions, including acute appendicitis or its complications. It did not have an on-call paediatric surgeon.

Josh was examined by the emergency department registrar, Dr Phillip Long, at 11:30 h. He obtained a history of abdominal pain, vomiting and decreased frequency of bowel motions. He thought that the vomiting had become faeculent. On examination, Josh was pale and unwell, having trouble ambulating, with a tachycardia of 103 bpm. There was generalised abdominal tenderness and guarding together with right iliac fossa tenderness and decreased bowel sounds. He ordered a full blood count, serum urea and electrolytes, CRP levels together with a plain x-ray of the abdomen. He inserted an intravenous cannula and administered fluids. The full blood count results came back showing an elevated white cell count of 10.9×10^9/L, a grossly elevated CRP level at 380 mg/L (reference <5 mg/L), decreased serum sodium and elevated serum potassium levels. The abdominal x-ray revealed dilated loops of small bowel consistent with small bowel obstruction, but no identifiable cause for the obstruction. Dr Long thought Josh needed to be transferred to the tertiary children's hospital for paediatric surgical review, but following protocol, paged the paediatric registrar on call to examine Josh. He informed the registrar that Josh was unwell, that his diagnosis was of bowel obstruction and that he needed to be transferred to a tertiary hospital for surgery.

Three hours after presentation, Josh was seen by the paediatric registrar, Dr Phoebe Feeney. Dr Feeney diagnosed Josh as having an acute abdomen secondary to bowel obstruction, the cause of which she could not state with any certainty. By this stage, Ed and Julie were very concerned about Josh's condition and the lack of progress that had been made, especially as Dr Sampson had already diagnosed acute appendicitis with possible rupture. Julie pleaded with Dr Feeney to order an ultrasound or CT scan of the abdomen to check whether Josh had acute appendicitis. Dr Feeney emphatically told Julie that she knew what the problem was and it was bowel obstruction and nothing to do with acute appendicitis. She told Julie that she was the doctor and not Julie.

Once Dr Feeney examined Josh, she formed the view that he needed to be seen by a paediatric surgeon. As there were no paediatric surgeons at the hospital, Josh needed to be transferred to the nearest tertiary referral children's hospital. Dr Long had been recommending the same thing for three hours. He felt, however, that the decision could not be made without paediatric review.

Josh was transferred to the tertiary hospital at 16:30 h on 12 May 2011 by the paediatric emergency transfer service. The retrieval team had told Dr Long to continue with the intravenous therapy, but at a higher rate. They also recommended intravenous antibiotics, which were commenced about 30 minutes prior to the arrival of the retrieval team.

About one hour after leaving the first hospital, Josh and his parents arrived at the paediatric emergency department at the tertiary hospital. Within 60 minutes, the paediatric surgical team saw Josh. They promptly diagnosed him as having acute appendicitis with a perforated appendix. Nonetheless, they ordered an abdominal ultrasound to see if there was any other problem. They also considered that Josh was dehydrated and not fit for surgery because of inadequate fluid resuscitation prior to his arrival. They ordered a bolus dose of normal saline with maintenance therapy of 500 mL at 108 mL/hr. They booked Josh in for surgery later that evening.

Two and a half hours after presentation, Josh underwent an abdominal ultrasound, which unsurprisingly demonstrated acute appendicitis, a perforated appendix and marked free fluid within the pelvis.

Five and a half hours after he presented to the tertiary hospital, Josh finally was taken to theatre. He first underwent a laparoscopic appendicectomy, but because of the perforation and obvious peritonitis, he proceeded to an open appendicectomy with washout of the peritoneal cavity.

After the operation, Josh was transferred to the ward rather than the paediatric intensive care unit (PICU). At about 04:00 h on 13 May 2011, Josh was reviewed by the paediatric registrar, who thought he was well-hydrated and made no further management orders. Two and a half hours later, he was again reviewed by the paediatric registrar, who changed his opinion and thought that Josh had septic shock with third spacing of fluid, electrolyte disturbances and dehydration. He ordered a fluid bolus and intravenous antibiotics and asked the PICU registrar to examine Josh. The paediatric surgical team then examined Josh and gave further orders of aliquots of normal saline, monitoring of urine output and antibiotics. He was finally transferred to PICU in the afternoon of 13 May 2011.

At about 24:00 h on 13 May 2011, Josh suffered a cardiac arrest from which he was resuscitated. The surgical team was called and attended urgently. Josh was rushed to theatre at about 01:30 h on 14 May 2011, where he underwent a laparotomy. Josh suffered another cardiac arrest during the surgery and could not be resuscitated.

LEGAL ISSUES

Ed and Julie commenced nervous shock proceedings against the first hospital and the tertiary children's hospital. They claimed that they had developed psychiatric conditions as a result of experiencing their son's death and the appalling treatment he had undergone.

A coronial inquest was conducted into Josh's death. The coroner found that he died as a result of a cardiac arrest caused by septic and/or hypovolaemic shock secondary to a ruptured appendix and acute peritonitis. He found that the diagnosis of acute appendicitis should have been made at presentation to the first hospital and acted upon.

Both Ed and Julie were devastated by Josh's death and what they saw to be gross failures in his care. They went so far as to state that the hospitals had murdered their son. They developed post-traumatic stress disorder and major depression. They were unable to continue working. None of these facts was disputed by the defendants.

Ed and Julie relied on the opinion of emergency department physicians, paediatricians and paediatric surgeons. Given the inquest, there ultimately was little dispute about the cause of Josh's death. The coroner's findings were that Josh's death was an avoidable tragedy. Fatal appendicitis is extremely rare in a developed country. It only occurs with delay in diagnosis, perforation, inadequate fluid replacement and inadequate control of sepsis. This all occurred in Josh's case. The experts agreed that his death was the direct consequence of a delay in diagnosis, inadequate resuscitation, a delay in antibiotic treatment and a delay in surgery.

Ed and Julie specifically drew attention to the management at the first hospital. They alleged that the hospital wrongly held itself out as providing general paediatric surgical services when it did not have that capacity. The ambulance service and local general practitioners were therefore misled about what services could be provided at the hospital. It effectively acted as a triage service for paediatrics, the surgical cases being transferred to another facility. As a consequence of this flawed system, there was a significant delay in getting Josh to the only hospital where surgery could be performed. It also resulted in his receiving inadequate assessment, inadequate resuscitation and delayed antibiotic therapy. By the time he arrived at the tertiary hospital, he was not in a fit state to undergo immediate surgery.

Dr Long should have made a diagnosis of acute appendicitis and rupture at 11:30 h on 12 May 2011. This was the same diagnosis made by the referring general practitioner, Dr Sampson. Dr Long knew that there was no surgeon on call and that there needed to be transfer to the tertiary hospital. But none of this occurred for hours. Julie pleaded with staff to perform an ultrasound (which was later performed at the tertiary referral hospital). An ultrasound may have accelerated treatment, although there was no evidence that this occurred at the tertiary referral hospital. In days gone-by a competent clinician could diagnose acute appendicitis without the use of an ultrasound. It is unfortunate that confirmation of the diagnosis was delayed pending ultrasound scanning.

At the inquest, it was the first hospital's emergency department's view that it was appropriate to bring emergency cases to the hospital's emergency department as it was more likely than general practitioners to be able to triage urgent cases accurately and then decide which cases needed to go to the tertiary referral hospital. As events turned out, this view was wrong. It was a patriarchal and arrogant view.

Ed and Julie's claims were settled at mediation.

Discussion

This avoidable tragedy highlights a number of important issues. First, it again highlights the importance doctors should attach to histories provided by parents of sick children. Parents intuitively know when their children are seriously unwell. They should not be fobbed off as appears to have been the case with Dr Feeney. If Dr Feeney had listened to Julie, she may have ordered an ultrasound, which would have shown acute appendicitis, perforation and acute peritonitis. Even if she were wedded to a diagnosis of bowel obstruction, she could not ascertain the cause of the bowel obstruction without further investigation. Her dismissive approach to both Josh's family and to Dr Long was unfortunate.

Secondly, blind adherence to protocols may not always be in the interest of patients. Doctors are trained to think rather than be automatons. Staff at the first hospital should not have required much assistance in arriving at the correct diagnosis and deciding to transfer Josh to the tertiary hospital. Dr Sampson had already provided the diagnosis to them in the referring letter. Why this was not acted upon earlier remained a mystery. Even if a diagnosis of bowel obstruction was relevant, no one thought to consider the cause. Josh clearly had bowel obstruction because the x-ray demonstrated this to be the case. In addition, he had not passed any motions and was thought to have vomited up faeculent material. The question was not whether he had bowel obstruction (as this was obvious), but what was the cause of the bowel obstruction.

More respect should be given to referring doctors by specialists, including trainee specialists in an emergency department or, as in this case, in paediatrics. General practitioners may have had years of experience in dealing with acutely unwell children. Dr Sampson's opinion was largely overlooked. He wished Josh to receive urgent paediatric surgical services. Instead, Josh received a deficient review by an emergency department registrar and a further deficient and delayed review by a paediatric registrar. Josh received none of the services for which he had been referred to the hospital.

Third, the case highlights a systemic problem in hospitals holding themselves out as offering certain services or facilities when they do not. There was no advantage at all in Josh being taken to the first hospital when it could not provide acute paediatric surgical services. The double handling of his assessment simply delayed his receiving adequate resuscitation and surgery. It led to his becoming so unstable that he was unable to cope with the first operation at the tertiary referral hospital.

Finally, the case highlights the importance of professional courtesy. In this case, there was no question of the paediatric registrar having significantly greater expertise than the emergency department registrar in the assessment of children. Dr Long's deference to her experience may have been warranted. The attitude of Dr Feeney was one of belittlement and discourtesy. Dr Long would not have requested an urgent examination if he did not feel that it was necessary. Unless there were pressing, urgent issues in the paediatrics ward, there was no reason for Dr Feeney to delay attending. Without respectful, civil communication, patient welfare may be put at risk.

Bullies exist in all workplaces. Their behaviour cannot be accepted. Policies or protocols need to be put in place in all medical workplaces to enable staff to feel safe and to give them a proper avenue to complain knowing that the process will be objective and fair. It goes without saying that doctors should not communicate in an arrogant or humiliating fashion to patients or family members, even appreciating that some situations are stressful and that sometimes family members can behave poorly as a result of that stress.

Clinical Principles

Acute appendicitis is a common reason for presentation in primary healthcare facilities, whether at an emergency department or in a general practice. In children, the consequences of a delay in diagnosis or a delay in diagnosing a perforated appendix can be catastrophic. Peritonitis can result in third spacing and dehydration. Children can rapidly decompensate if they do not receive proper intravenous therapy and early intervention. Acute appendicitis is not some benign condition where a simple appendicectomy is all that is required. It should be treated seriously and urgently.

OBESITY

History

Sebastian Lopez was diagnosed with liver cancer in September 2011 at the age of 67. He thought that his cancer was due to exposure to toxic chemicals while working as a cleaner in the 1980s. The liver cancer was, in fact, caused by his obesity. Sebastian had been obese for many years. While he knew that obesity was not good for his health, it came as a surprise to be told that his obesity could damage his liver and ultimately lead to hepatocellular carcinoma (HCC).

From 1997 until 2011, Dr Felix Garcia was Sebastian's general practitioner. He consulted Dr Garcia because one aspect of his medical practice was environmental medicine. Sebastian thought that this specialisation was relevant given his concern about being exposed to toxic substances in the workplace.

When he first consulted Dr Garcia, Sebastian weighed 140 kg, suffered from obstructive sleep apnoea (OSA), maturity onset diabetes mellitus, hypertension and the metabolic syndrome. He had not worked since 1992. He had respiratory problems, back and knee pain secondary to his obesity and a five-year history of abnormal liver function tests (LFTs). He had attended a tertiary referral hospital obesity and diabetic clinic and had been advised many times to lose weight. On occasions, he had lost significant weight, but he always put it back on. Conservative measures to treat his obesity had therefore failed. By the time of his first consultation with Sebastian, Dr Garcia was aware of Sebastian's medical history, including his inability to achieve sustained weight loss.

Early in their therapeutic relationship, in 1997, Dr Garcia ordered a number of blood tests, including LFTs. There was elevation of alkaline phosphatase (ALP 137 U/L, reference 30–115 U/L), alanine aminotransferase (ALT 56 U/L, reference <55 U/L), aspartate aminotransferase (AST 46 U/L, reference <40 U/L) and gamma glutamyl transferase (GGT 137 U/L, reference <60 U/L). His serum albumin was 37 g/L (reference 38–55 g/L). Dr Garcia diagnosed Sebastian with a fatty liver.

Dr Garcia thereafter ordered regular LFTs and received the results of LFTs ordered at various hospitals or specialists Sebastian had visited. The LFTs were persistently elevated. Sebastian's serum albumin was 29 g/L in 1998. The albumin level was normal in 1999, but was low thereafter. The transaminases remained elevated and the albumin remained low from 2000.

In May 1999, Dr Garcia diagnosed Sebastian as having cholestatic hepatitis based upon the abnormal LFTs and an ultrasound suggesting gallstones. There was however no evidence of bile duct obstruction.

Later in 1999, Dr Garcia diagnosed Sebastian as suffering from metronidazole-induced cholestatic hepatitis, even though the LFTs had been abnormal for a number of years. He referred Sebastian to a gastroenterologist, who thought that the abdominal pain was secondary to gallstones and referred Sebastian to a gastrointestinal surgeon. The surgeon referred Sebastian to a dietitian.

In 2000, Sebastian underwent a laparoscopic cholecystectomy at a different tertiary referral hospital from the first. Despite having his gallbladder removed, Sebastian's LFTs remained abnormal.

He developed ascites and signs of portal hypertension, and was diagnosed with micronodular cirrhosis and liver failure in 2003 after a liver biopsy at a third tertiary referral hospital.

His liver disease was regularly monitored at a fourth tertiary referral hospital in the same city. In 2011, he underwent a CT scan and ultrasound, which demonstrated HCC.

Legal Issues

Sebastian commenced proceedings against Dr Garcia in the state Supreme Court in 2012. He alleged, among other things, that Dr Garcia breached his duty of care by failing to refer him to a hepatologist in light of his long-standing abnormal LFTs, and for failing to refer him directly to a bariatric surgeon for advice about bariatric surgery given the fact that conservative measures to overcome his obesity had failed.

The case was complicated by the fact that Dr Garcia advised Sebastian that his abnormal LFTs were the consequence of his workplace exposure to toxic chemicals and metals. Dr Garcia had been an expert witness in proceedings against Sebastian's former employer for exposure to chemicals. That case had failed.

Expert evidence was called from general practitioners, hepatologists, bariatric surgeons and endocrinologists. Sebastian succeeded at first instance. In a decision published in 2012, the judge found that Dr Garcia breached his duty of care by failing to refer Sebastian to a hepatologist by September 2000, and by failing to refer him directly to a bariatric surgeon.

Bariatric surgery was reserved for patients who had tried to lose weight by conservative (medical) means and had demonstrably failed. The trial judge found that Sebastian eminently qualified for consideration of bariatric surgery. If a patient had lost weight in the past and then regained it, and was seriously obese with comorbidities, then he should be offered surgery.

There was no question in the proceedings that, if Sebastian's liver problems had been properly investigated, he would have been referred to a hepatologist and undergone a liver biopsy. He would have been diagnosed with nonalcoholic steatohepatitis (NASH). There was an argument at trial as to whether he had cirrhosis from 1997 when he first consulted Dr Garcia. Once a person has cirrhosis, bariatric surgery is unlikely to be offered. The expert bariatric surgical opinion was that, if the diagnosis was confined to NASH, then bariatric surgery would have halted the progression of the underlying disease and Sebastian would not have developed cirrhosis or liver cancer.

There was a significant backlash from general practitioner groups after the judgment. They were outraged by a result they perceived as making a general practitioner liable for a patient's obesity. Of course, the case was not about that at all. It was about how obesity should be managed, especially once a complication like NASH develops. The view that it is largely the patient's fault is fast becoming outdated.

Dr Garcia appealed. In 2013, the state Court of Appeal allowed the appeal and entered judgment for Dr Garcia. The trial judge's finding that Dr Garcia breached his duty of care by failing to refer Sebastian to a hepatologist was not disputed or overturned on appeal. The Court of Appeal overturned the trial judge's decision that Sebastian ought to have been directly referred to a bariatric surgeon. There was no convincing evidence that general practitioners at the time would routinely refer morbidly obese patients to a bariatric surgeon, rather than give advice to lose weight or refer the patient to an obesity clinic.

Sebastian lost his case because he could not prove causation: he could not prove that he would have undergone bariatric surgery if referred to a hepatologist earlier. There was a difference of opinion among the expert hepatologists called in the case about whether a hypothetical reasonable hepatologist would have simply advised Sebastian to lose weight, sent him to an obesity clinic or referred him to a bariatric surgeon. Sebastian was unable to establish that he probably would have been referred to a bariatric surgeon if he had been referred to a hepatologist in 1999 or 2000.

The bariatric surgeons in the case agreed that Sebastian would have been offered bariatric surgery if he had been referred earlier. Sebastian simply could not prove that he would have been referred before he developed cirrhosis.

Sebastian sought special leave to appeal to the High Court. Special leave was refused. Sebastian died in 2015.

Discussion

This case highlights the gravity of the obesity epidemic in the Australian community. Obesity is a serious medical condition of complex aetiology. It is associated with disabling comorbidities, including diabetes, musculoskeletal problems, obstructive sleep apnoea and liver disease. Sebastian suffered from all of these secondary problems. Obesity is a difficult condition to treat. It is not a simple matter of advising a patient to lose weight. Dietary measures have mixed success. What is essential is the provision of proper advice and information about obesity, the risks associated with it and the need for a multidisciplinary approach to therapy. As here, sometimes treatment may involve bariatric surgeons and hepatologists. A one-size-fits-all approach is unlikely to achieve long-term success.

The case also highlights a medical blind spot. While Dr Garcia appreciated that Sebastian had fatty liver disease at the outset, he failed to appreciate that the persistently abnormal LFTs could be associated with the obesity. He diagnosed extrahepatic cholestasis and a metronidazole-induced illness or toxicity secondary to workplace exposures to chemicals.

The reason for the abnormal LFTs was always there in front of him: obesity. As a result of this blind spot, Sebastian was not diagnosed with NASH until 2003, when he already had micronodular cirrhosis of the liver and liver failure. His nonalcoholic fatty liver disease progressed to NASH and then to cirrhosis with liver failure. Patients with cirrhosis are at an increased risk of HCC. Sebastian unfortunately developed HCC as well.

It may have been reasonable initially to look for other causes for the persistent derangement of the LFTs, such as gallstones. However, after cholecystectomy, extrahepatic cholestatic hepatitis could not reasonably be considered the cause. Sebastian did not at any time have evidence of dilation of his common bile duct or any other duct in the biliary tree. His cholestatic pattern of abnormal LFTs reflected hepatocellular injury and intrinsic small duct obstruction due to inflammation and fibrosis.

Without first investigating and excluding other possible causes of Sebastian's persistently abnormal LFTs, Dr Garcia should not have assumed they were caused by workplace exposure to chemicals and metals.

The case also highlighted the negative attitude towards obese patients, such as the perception that fault lies with a patient for eating too much, or that if a patient ignores a general practitioner's advice to lose weight, then there is nothing more to be done.

Clinical Principles

The management of obesity and liver dysfunction requires thoughtful coordination of care. Obesity is a risk factor for deranged LFTs, inflammation and fibrosis of the liver and liver cancer.

A general practitioner is in the ideal position to coordinate treatment of obesity. This may be a long and complex process.

ABDOMINAL PAIN

History

In September 2011 at the age of 36, Liz Chadwick developed severe, right-sided, colicky, lower abdominal pain. Her general practitioner, concerned about a possible ectopic pregnancy or acute appendicitis, referred her to the emergency department at the nearest private hospital. Investigations excluded both an ectopic pregnancy and acute appendicitis. The pain was eased by analgesia, and Liz was discharged home with a prescription for analgesics.

The pain persisted. Five days after being discharged from the emergency department, Liz consulted her general practitioner again, who referred her to the emergency department of a private hospital. The pain by this time had changed location and was now localised to the right upper quadrant. It was aggravated by lying flat, and was associated with nausea and vomiting. Staff at the hospital did not consider there was any significant pathology and discharged Liz back into the care of her general practitioner with a further prescription for analgesics.

About six weeks later, Liz again consulted her general practitioner complaining of abdominal pain. He referred her to a different private hospital emergency department. The history recorded was of nausea and vomiting, some diarrhoea, and epigastric abdominal pain radiating to the left side of the abdomen for 48 hours; and episodic vomiting for six months.

An ultrasound of the upper abdomen was performed, which demonstrated multiple calculi in the gallbladder and gallbladder wall thickening, but no dilation of the biliary tree. A CT scan of the abdomen and pelvis demonstrated diffuse gallbladder wall thickening and stranding around the pancreas consistent with acute pancreatitis or acute cholecystitis with secondary stranding of the pancreas. Blood tests revealed gross elevations of serum amylase and serum lipase (markers of acute pancreatitis), and abnormal LFTs.

While in the emergency department, general surgeon Dr Frank Briggs was asked to review Liz. He made a diagnosis of acute pancreatitis secondary to cholelithiasis (gallstones) and recommended surgery to remove Liz's gall bladder a week later, once the inflammation had settled. Liz consented to the operation. She remained nil by mouth, and was administered intravenous fluids, analgesia and antibiotics. Dr Briggs did not give her any warnings about the risk of bile duct injury associated with the operation, or of the magnitude of the risk, or of the potential consequences if the bile duct would be injured.

A week later, the serum markers of acute pancreatitis and the abnormal liver function had improved significantly. Liz proceeded to laparoscopic cholecystectomy as planned.

During the procedure, Dr Briggs attempted an intraoperative cholangiogram (IOC) to define the biliary tree. He was unable to do so because the cystic duct was too narrow to be cannulated. Dr Briggs's operative findings were of a normal gallbladder with no evidence of acute cholecystitis. He found no evidence of pancreatitis. His operative diagnosis for Liz's prior presentations was acute on chronic cholecystitis. Histopathological examination of the resected gallbladder later showed a thickened wall and chronic inflammation. Dr Briggs's operative note was "routine chole". These facts were contained in correspondence to Liz's general practitioner, well after her operation.

On the day after the laparoscopic cholecystectomy, Liz experienced significant abdominal pain with tachycardia, and pyrexia of 38.1°C. She required oxycodone 10 mg at 21:30 h and 22:00 h that evening, tramadol at 04:30 h the next morning and further oxycodone at 07:30 h and 12:10 h. Her abdominal pain and fever continued.

Notwithstanding her symptoms and signs, Dr Briggs discharged her from the hospital on the fourth postoperative day. She consulted her general practitioner later that day because of her pain. He ordered a plain abdominal x-ray, which demonstrated multiple clips in the right upper quadrant, and a CT scan of the abdomen, which showed extensive free fluid in the abdominal cavity and pelvis and around the liver, consistent with acute peritonitis and infection. A full blood count demonstrated a neutrophil (11.5×10^9/L, reference 1.5–8.0 $\times 10^9$/L) leucocytosis (13.2×10^9/L, reference 4.5–11.0 $\times 10^9$/L), and a grossly elevated CRP (240 mg/L, reference <5.0 mg/L). The serum amylase and lipase levels were normal.

After the CT scan, Liz was referred back to the emergency department at the private hospital, where she was reviewed by Dr Briggs. Dr Briggs considered she was suffering from another episode of pancreatitis. He thought she needed an endoscopic retrograde cholangiopancreatogram (ERCP) to ascertain whether there was a stone blocking the pancreatic duct. He arranged transfer to a tertiary referral hospital for the test.

After the ERCP, Liz was examined by an upper gastrointestinal tract (GIT) surgeon, Dr Ernest Fleming, who diagnosed her with biliary peritonitis secondary to a leak from the cystic duct stump. At laparoscopy, Dr Fleming repaired the leaking duct, drained 2.5 L of bile-stained fluid from her abdomen, and inserted a drain into the area. Liz gradually improved, but still complained of abdominal and pelvic pain, and bloating. She was anxious about the possibilities of infertility and bowel obstruction.

LEGAL ISSUES

Liz commenced proceedings in negligence against Dr Briggs for failing to warn her of the risk of bile duct injury, failing to identify the biliary anatomy adequately and, in consequence, failing to ligate the cystic duct during the cholecystectomy. She also alleged that Dr Briggs failed promptly to diagnose biliary peritonitis and to take steps to repair the leaking cystic duct.

Liz relied on the opinions of a general surgeon and an upper GIT surgeon. Dr Briggs relied on the opinions of a general surgeon, who maintained that the performance of the cholecystectomy was in accordance with acceptable standards with the cystic duct injury being no more than the materialisation of an inherent risk of such surgery that might happen even in the best of hands. He also considered that earlier diagnosis of biliary peritonitis would not have altered Liz's outcome.

Liz's experts disputed these arguments, although conceded that earlier diagnosis and treatment of the biliary peritonitis would not have materially changed her long-term condition.

The matter went to mediation and was resolved on confidential terms.

Discussion

There was no issue that the cholecystectomy was properly indicated.

Thus, the first issue that arose was whether Liz was warned about the risk of bile duct injury and its consequences. She asserted that she had not been warned. There was no contemporaneous record indicating that she had been warned. The consent form she signed made no mention of bile duct injury. Nonetheless, Dr Briggs in his defence to proceedings claimed that, in accordance with his usual practice, he would no doubt have warned Liz of the risk of bile duct injury.

While this case emphasises the importance of providing adequate information to a patient to enable proper consent to a procedure, it also highlights how, at a practical legal level, a failure to warn case is rarely prosecuted successfully.

There was a dispute about whether a warning was given. It was unlikely Liz would have succeeded with this claim at trial. Firstly, a court usually does not accept subjective circumstantial evidence of a plaintiff given in hindsight suggesting that consent would not have been given for the procedure if there had been appropriate warnings of the risks. Indeed, evidence of what an injured plaintiff would have done if warned of a risk of injury is often inadmissible.

Secondly, and although not relevant to Liz's case, there is often a contemporaneous medical record noting that a warning was given. A court generally gives significant weight to a contemporaneous record of the provision of a warning and a discussion of its import.

Thirdly, and most importantly, a plaintiff must prove that she would not have undergone the operation and suffered the injury that arose if warned appropriately. Here, Liz had significant pain that resulted in multiple presentations. Even if she were warned of the small risk of bile duct injury and its ramifications, she was likely to have still gone ahead with the operation because of the disabling nature of her pain and the need to have it remedied.

The central issue in the case concerned the correct identification of the relevant structures during the laparoscopic cholecystectomy. As is usual for cases involving possible intraoperative negligence, whether there was incompetence in the performance of the operation leading to bile duct injury is a matter of inference, in the absence of an incriminating note in the operation record, progress notes or postoperative correspondence of the surgeon.

Dr Briggs's handwritten operation note did not include a record of any problems encountered during the procedure. The typed operation note also did not include a reference to any problem encountered during the procedure. Dr Briggs's correspondence with Liz's general practitioner did not contain any admission of error. Although absence of admission or error does not exclude negligence, such absence often makes it very difficult to establish negligence.

There are a number of pieces of evidence that may point to intraoperative negligence, including expert evidence about the anatomy of the area of the operation, expert evidence about the usual way in which the operation is performed, the postoperative course of the patient and the nature of the complication ultimately diagnosed.

In order to remove the gallbladder, it is necessary to identify the cystic duct entering the gallbladder. A proximal clip is then placed on the cystic duct close to the gallbladder and an IOC performed. There is a debate in the scientific literature about whether an IOC is necessary. Once the biliary tree architecture and any stones have been demonstrated, a clip is placed distally on the cystic duct at or below the level of dissection. The duct is then cut between the clips and the gallbladder is removed.

It is important for any surgeon removing the gallbladder to be cognisant of the anatomy of the biliary tree (hepatic ducts, cystic duct, common bile duct). If an IOC is not used, or is unable to be performed, as here, then identification of the anatomy is achieved by adequate dissection and direct inspection. Here, Dr Briggs found that the cystic duct was small and could not be cannulated. The bile leak was identified eventually as coming from the cystic duct stump. It is difficult to see how a biliary leak could occur from a cystic duct if it had been adequately identified and properly ligated in the first place.

Given the unusual number of clips applied in the vicinity of the cystic duct, it may be inferred that Dr Briggs experienced difficulties during the operation. In the circumstances, proper practice required the insertion of a drain during the operation. If a drain had been inserted then, according to the expert evidence, a biliary leak would have been observed in the immediate postoperative period. The drain would have been left in situ until the hole in the cystic duct had healed. Liz would not have required any further operations. She would have avoided biliary peritonitis.

In Liz's case the symptoms and signs of biliary peritonitis manifested early in the postoperative period. This suggested that the cystic duct had never been adequately clipped. If the clips had dislodged or slipped over time, then there would have been a more gradual onset of Liz's pain, tachycardia and pyrexia.

Finally, Dr Briggs's operation note was, at best, succinct. It was likely to be easier for a court to draw inferences of probable negligence against him when he did not take the time to record his operation in a professional manner.

Clinical Principles

Dr Briggs failed to document adequately the details of his operation. If he had done so, he may have better assessed the postoperative course, and recognised the biliary leak.

In addition, once the IOC failed, he ought to have been aware that correct identification of the biliary anatomy required meticulous dissection and visualisation. There was no evidence that he took additional care with this part of the operation. The use of many staples in the area of operation and the fact that a leak occurred imply a less than ideal dissection.

At the time of operation, he might have consulted an experienced colleague to discuss management of the difficulties he had encountered in identifying and securing the cystic duct, and sought physical assistance if required.

UNEXPLAINED WEIGHT LOSS

History

Steve Coates was a 24-year-old, fit and healthy Indigenous Australian, who lived in a rural community. He was in a long-term relationship with Amber, with whom he had a young daughter, Taylor, to support. Steve was a professional rugby league player and hoped to obtain a contract with one of the state capital rugby league clubs in the future.

In June 2006, Steve presented to his general practitioner with unexplained weight loss and a three-month history of loose motions. During football season he usually weighed 102 kg. His weight had dropped to 73 kg. Some of his bowel motions were mixed with mucus and blood. Although Amber was supportive of his career, there was frequent tension in their relationship. Steve also worried about how he was going to provide for his family given the difficulties of earning an income as a professional rugby league player in a regional centre.

His general practitioner, Dr Geoff Rowley, thought the weight loss was due to a hard preseason training regime. He thought the gastrointestinal symptoms were caused by an infective enteritis, inflammatory bowel disease or irritable bowel syndrome. He referred Steve to the local general physician, Dr Jack Fairweather, for advice and treatment.

Steve saw Dr Fairweather two days later. He obtained a similar history to that obtained by Dr Rowley. He noted that blood was mixed in bowel motions and that Steve experienced increased flatulence. Despite the weight loss, Steve reported not having any difficulties keeping up with the football team at training or during games. On abdominal examination, Dr Fairweather found no abnormalities. He did not perform a rectal examination. He did not order a faecal occult blood (FOB) test, microscopy and culture of a stool sample or any other test. Dr Fairweather diagnosed Steve as having an infective colitis of some type and prescribed metronidazole. He advised Steve that if the metronidazole did not work then there may be a need for a colonoscopy and multiple biopsies of the colon because of the possibility of an inflammatory bowel disease such as ulcerative colitis.

About a month later (August 2006), Steve again presented to his general practitioner for advice about continued weight loss and changes in his bowel habit. He had lost additional weight, and still complained of flatulence and blood mixed in his motions. The episodes of loose bowel motions fluctuated with periods of constipation. Dr Rowley telephoned Dr Fairweather, who suggested a further course of metronidazole. He also suggested that there might be a disaccharidase deficiency and advised Dr Rowley to tell Steve to avoid milk products. A stool sample was not considered necessary. On examination, Dr Rowley found a mass in the left inguinal fossa. He thought Steve had a "loaded colon", presumably because of the episodes of constipation. Steve bluntly asked Dr Rowley whether he had bowel cancer. Dr Rowley said that it was very unlikely in light of his age, but ordered no investigation to confirm or exclude the disease or to justify his opinion.

Steve returned to his general practitioner the next month. He had lost further weight and, according to the clinical record of the general practitioner, looked "very lean". Steve wanted to have an ultrasound to ascertain what was going on in his abdomen. Instead, the general practitioner telephoned Dr Fairweather, who suggested that Dr Rowley order some blood tests to exclude coeliac disease. Dr Rowley did as instructed, but the tests failed to reveal any abnormality suggestive of coeliac disease.

In October 2006, Steve telephoned his general practitioner, asking for a further appointment with Dr Fairweather. He complained of abdominal pain, especially after large meals, and felt that his abdomen was distended. He had lost his appetite and his weight had dropped further. In addition, he still complained of blood and mucus in his bowel movements, which fluctuated between constipation and diarrhoea. Dr Rowley organised a consultation with Dr Fairweather the next day.

Dr Fairweather confirmed the history provided to Dr Rowley. He also noted on further interrogation that the episodes of abdominal discomfort and bloating were not related to any particular type of food. Dr Fairweather advised Steve that it was difficult to make a diagnosis in circumstances where Steve was under financial and relationship stress. He ordered an upper abdominal ultrasound, LFTs, a full blood count (FBC) and inflammatory marker (ESR and CRP) levels . Dr Fairweather raised the possibility of Steve's needing an upper small bowel biopsy looking for a disaccharidase deficiency if the ordered tests were normal.

The ultrasound of the upper abdomen was normal. A full blood count demonstrated mild anaemia (126 g/L, reference 130–180 g/L). All other tests were normal.

Steve returned to see Dr Fairweather two weeks after the tests to discuss the results. Dr Fairweather diagnosed a mild depression and reassured Steve that there was "nothing serious going on". He advised him to avoid milk products to see whether he had a lactose intolerance.

One month later, soon before Christmas 2006, Steve returned to see Dr Fairweather because of increased abdominal pain. Dr Fairweather encouraged Steve to lift his mood and counselled him about the difficulties with his career and his relationship.

The problems of intermittent abdominal pain, bloating, variable bowel motions and blood and mucus mixed in with bowel motions continued for a number of months. Steve assumed his problems were due to stress and endeavoured to manage it as best he could.

He continued to lose weight despite eating well. He was referred back to see Dr Fairweather in May 2007. At the time of the consultation, Steve's weight had dropped to 68 kg. Dr Fairweather diagnosed depression and irritable bowel syndrome. He prescribed an antidepressant, doxepin, 25 mg at night, and represcribed metronidazole on the basis that there may be some residual colitis.

Later that month, Dr Rowley ordered a FBC and iron studies. These showed a microcytic hypochromic anaemia consistent with an iron deficiency due to chronic blood loss. The test results were copied to Dr Fairweather. Notwithstanding the results and Steve's symptoms, no FOB test was ordered. No abdominal or digital rectal examination was performed, and no arrangement was made for a colonoscopy.

Irritable bowel syndrome and depression remained the operative diagnoses throughout May and most of June 2007.

Early in the morning on 30 June 2007, Steve presented to the emergency department at the local base hospital with a two-week history of increasingly severe, colicky abdominal pain associated with bloating. He recounted the history he had provided to Dr Fairweather and Dr Rowley over the preceding 12 months. The emergency department specialist noted that Steve had not undergone a colonoscopy. He found lower abdominal tenderness and a palpable left inguinal mass. A tender mass was also palpable on digital rectal examination about 3 cm from the anus. His provisional diagnoses were rectal carcinoma and bowel obstruction. Arrangements were made for Steve to be seen urgently by a general surgeon that day. Blood tests ordered at the hospital demonstrated an iron deficiency anaemia. There was also a grossly elevated carcinoembryonic antigen level consistent with bowel cancer (288.4 ng/mL, reference <3.0 ng/mL).

The general surgeon ordered a CT scan of the abdomen, which showed circumferential thickening of the entire rectum up to the rectosigmoid junction. There was significant abdominal and pelvic ascites with thickening of the greater omentum, suggesting peritoneal seeding of the peritoneum. There was also a mass in the presacral space adjacent to the rectum, suggesting direct extension of the cancer. Partial bowel obstruction was evident. There was no sign of spread to the liver, bones or any other organ.

At laparoscopy on 30 June 2007, there were scattered peritoneal cancerous nodules and gross ascites. The surgeon converted the operation to a laparotomy and performed a defunctioning sigmoid loop colostomy to relieve the bowel obstruction. He was unable to resect the cancer. Histopathological analysis of the operative biopsy specimen demonstrated a mucin-secreting invasive adenocarcinoma of the rectum. Steve's rectal cancer was Duke's stage D (widespread metastases).

While in hospital, Steve developed obstruction of the left ureter as a result of direct invasion of the cancer. This resulted in a left hydronephrosis and the need for a cystoscopy and insertion of a ureteric stent.

The surgeon referred Steve to the medical oncology department at a city tertiary referral hospital. He underwent chemotherapy, but this was unsuccessful. Steve died in the early hours of 2 September 2008 in the local hospital where he was receiving terminal care.

Legal Issues

In 2011, Steve's father commenced proceedings against Dr Fairweather and Dr Rowley on behalf of Steve's daughter, Taylor. The proceedings were brought under the Compensation to Relatives Act 1897 (NSW) for Taylor's loss, as Steve's dependent, of the services (e.g. child care) and income she expected to receive from him had he survived. Steve's immediate family also sued Dr Fairweather for nervous shock, claiming they had developed psychiatric conditions including depression as a result of Steve's death.

It was alleged that Dr Fairweather should have performed a digital rectal examination and, more importantly, proceeded to a colonoscopy following Steve's first consultation with him in June 2006 and at all subsequent consultations.

Dr Fairweather admitted that he breached his duty of care to Steve (and Steve's family) by not taking steps that would have led to the diagnosis of rectal carcinoma as early as June 2006. However, he put causation in issue.

Steve's family sought the opinions of a gastroenterologist, medical oncologist and colorectal surgeon. Their collective view was that, in June 2006, Steve would have had a Duke's A or B cancer, which means it would have been a carcinoma in situ or a carcinoma that had not penetrated through the wall of the rectum. Steve would more likely than not have undergone resection of the cancer and survived. Even if the cancer had spread through the wall of the rectum (Duke's C), he would have undergone treatment with curative intent and more likely than not would have survived long-term.

The expert colorectal surgeon qualified by Dr Fairweather's solicitors argued that, although in June 2006, the rectal cancer would probably have been a Duke's B malignancy, there were also chances that it could have been Duke's A, C or D, and the weighted average of these chances meant that the likelihood of cure was only 30%. When analysed properly, the expert's opinion was very similar to those of the experts relied on by Steve's family.

Dr Rowley argued that, at all times, it was reasonable to rely on Dr Fairweather's advice and treatment as a specialist.

The claim was settled at mediation.

Discussion

This case highlights the importance of excluding a sinister condition before ascribing presenting symptoms to a benign or psychiatric condition.

At the time of Steve's first consultation with him, Dr Fairweather recognised the need to perform a colonoscopy, but this was never followed up. Instead, and despite Steve's weight loss and gastrointestinal symptoms worsening, Dr Fairweather diagnosed depression and irritable bowel syndrome. While Steve may well have suffered from depression, Dr Fairweather was never justified in diagnosing irritable bowel syndrome when he had not ordered any investigation or performed any procedure that was capable of excluding serious intestinal disease. Even when he diagnosed colitis at the first consultation in June 2006, Dr Fairweather failed to order any test to confirm his diagnosis.

There was no evidence that Dr Fairweather performed a mental state examination of Steve, or that the diagnosis of depression was appropriate. The dose of doxepin was probably not sufficient to be effective, even if it was the case that Steve required medication for depression. It may be that Dr Fairweather felt comfortable that he had prescribed something rather than nothing for Steve, even though the treatment may not have been appropriate.

Steve presented with all of the classical features of colorectal cancer. He had unexplained weight loss, blood in his motions and a change in bowel habit. The reasons for not taking Steve's obvious symptoms and signs seriously were unclear. Dr Fairweather's first impression may have been that Steve "looked well", perhaps because he was familiar with Steve's football career.

The symptoms and signs might have been ignored on the basis that Steve was either too young to have bowel cancer or that he was under stress and suffering from depression. Further, some of the investigations ordered by Dr Fairweather were illogical. For example, it is difficult to see how an ultrasound of the upper abdomen had anything to do with signs and symptoms localised to the lower abdomen, including bright blood in Steve's bowel movements.

Clinical Principles

This tragic case also highlights the importance of specialist opinions to the management of patients by general practitioners. Dr Fairweather's advice unquestionably coloured the treatment and investigations provided to Steve by Dr Rowley. Dr Rowley might have felt constrained by Dr Fairweather's opinion, especially in the context of practice in a rural town.

Primary health care providers, including country general practitioners, have an obligation to provide thoughtful and adequate diagnostic work-up for every patient. This will require referrals for specialist opinions in many instances, and may require multiple visits to arrange and review tests and opinions. Dr Rowley's lawyers attempted unsuccessfully to argue that pressure of work in the country somehow absolved Dr Rowley of his responsibility.

RECTAL BLEEDING

History

Harry Adams, aged 42 in 2002, attended a public hospital for haemorrhoidectomy. He had suffered from constipation, rectal bleeding and haemorrhoids for at least a decade. At the time of making a medicolegal complaint 11 years later, there was no detail available at the hospital of the preoperative clinical findings, or of the operative procedure, or of the identity of the surgeon.

In 2007 Harry presented to his then general practitioner because of testicular pain on sexual intercourse. At that consultation he also complained of "haemorrhoids". The record of the examination was brief, noting a large and tender left testicle and the presence of haemorrhoids, with no further examination detail. An ultrasound showed a mildly enlarged left testicle, with dimensions of 25 mm × 33 mm × 53 mm and a right testicle of normal size, being 24 mm × 31 mm × 24 mm. The radiologist diagnosed mild orchitis, and a small hydrocele.

Harry was prescribed a course of doxycycline and referred to a surgeon for management of his haemorrhoids. The referral letter was brief, merely stating that the reason for referral was "Piles Bleeding".

It was not until six months later in 2008 that Harry visited the surgeon, whose notes referred to three years of rectal bleeding for which, on one occasion two years previously, Harry had attended the local hospital because of excessive bleeding. There was no detail of management at the hospital.

The surgeon's notes stated that the family history was negative for bowel cancer and that Harry's general health was good. Clinical examination revealed chronically prolapsed haemorrhoids at the right anterior and right posterior positions. Sigmoidoscopy showed a large sessile rectal polyp on the right rectal wall.

Colonoscopy was performed at a private hospital the following week. This showed a mid rectal polyp 4 cm in length and two small (3–4 mm) colonic polyps. All were removed. Histopathology of the larger polyp demonstrated intramucosal adenocarcinoma. One of the two smaller polyps showed a mildly dysplastic tubular adenoma.

The surgeon sent a copy of the histopathology report to the referring practitioner and commented that he would be discussing the issues with Harry over the next few weeks, that he would continue to manage Harry, and that he would communicate with the referring practitioner about Harry's progress.

The surgeon gave two contradictory messages to the general practitioner. In an initial letter, prior to receipt of the histopathology, the surgeon suggested that an ultra-low anterior resection would be necessary if the lesion proved to be malignant. In his next letter, after receipt of the histopathology, he wrote that there was malignancy, and that the early invasive adenocarcinoma would be adequately managed with polypectomy and diligent follow-up.

The surgeon's notes did not refer to any conversation with Harry about the risks and benefits of different surgical approaches. At the time the complaint commenced, the surgeon had retired because of advanced age.

Since Harry's rectal bleeding had continued intermittently for nearly two decades, he decided that this was simply his lot, especially since he understood that he had received curative treatment for rectal cancer in 2008.

In 2010 Harry attended a second general practitioner (at a different clinic from the first general practitioner) because of occasional rectal bleeding. This second general practitioner noted that there had been a long history of intermittent rectal bleeding prior to the colonoscopy.

This general practitioner referred Harry to a consultant different from the previous one, with the request that he manage the rectal bleeding. Harry's partner contacted the previous surgeon's rooms immediately, requesting that a copy of the histopathology report be faxed to the new general practitioner's clinic. One hour following the consultation the clinic received a fax confirming the presence of an adenocarcinoma. Neither the second general practitioner nor anyone else at the clinic contacted Harry or the surgeon to whom Harry had been referred to discuss the findings.

The letter to the second surgeon referred to the original investigation in the following terms, "Colonoscopy – normal?" This was the case as far as this practitioner understood it to be at the time of seeing Harry; it was not the case on receipt of the fax one hour later. In the event, Harry did not consult with the second surgeon.

Nearly a year later in 2011 Harry attended the second general practice clinic again, this time because of his desire to quit smoking. He saw a third general practitioner. A prescription was written for varenicline, without any advice about possible side effects. There was no reference to Harry's bowel disorder.

Six months later Harry saw a third doctor, at the latter general practice clinic, because of an eye infection. The next week Harry saw the original doctor from that practice, for a pertussis vaccination. There was no record of discussion of the bowel problem or of the histopathology result.

General practitioner number four saw the patient four times over two years, on the last occasion because of altered bowel habit. At that consultation in 2012 the doctor reviewed the notes and discovered the histopathology result of four years previously.

The colonoscopy that followed this latest consultation demonstrated a fungating rectal tumour. Two days following the colonoscopy Harry experienced increasing and debilitating abdominal pain that led to hospital admission and investigation. The neutrophil count was 8.6×10^9/L (reference 1.5–8.0×10^9/L) and the gamma glutamyl transferase was 154 U/L (reference 8–64 U/L). Inflammatory markers, ESR and CRP, were not performed. The cause of the recent pain was not determined, and Harry was discharged home.

An outpatient PET (positron emission tomogram) scan demonstrated a hypermetabolic mass in the rectum extending into the surrounding fat, involving regional lymph nodes, the left pelvis, the paracaval region and most of both lobes of the liver.

A consultant surgeon attached to the latter hospital saw Harry one week following discharge and referred him for radiation therapy. Two months later a surveillance CT of the abdomen was performed. This revealed free gas within the peritoneal cavity. Presumably rectal perforation was the cause of debilitating pain two months previously.

Harry passed away six days following the CT scan. The final diagnosis was stage four metastatic colorectal carcinoma and a perforated bowel.

Legal Issues

In 2013 Harry's partner sought compensation for the consequences of delayed investigation and treatment. She was concerned that there were several opportunities to effectively address Harry's problem. Because of poor management in different clinics, these opportunities were lost.

Although the 2008 histopathologic findings had been successfully sourced on request in 2010, the 2008 private hospital file had been destroyed when Harry's partner commenced proceedings in 2013.

The matter is ongoing.

Discussion

The first thing to consider is the legislative requirement for the retention of medical records. For an adult in the state where this clinical problem occurred, the law mandates that records be retained for seven years from the date of the last consultation or procedure and, in the case of children, until the child turns 25. If Harry's earlier records had been available, the analysis of his clinical problem would have been simpler.

Record retention problems such as this are likely to become less of an issue in time, as most general practitioners, medical consultants, other health professionals and hospitals now maintain electronic records. Also, electronic general practice records are sometimes available at the local referral hospital, and vice versa. A strong case can be made to use personal patient-retained health records.

It is unknown what clinical assessment occurred at the time of initial haemorrhoidectomy, but it is likely that a detailed examination of the rectum was performed. When Harry saw the surgeon five years later, the rectal mass was 4 cm in length. If this had been a slow-growing tumour, it is possible that the rectum was not normal in 2002 (at the time of haemorrhoidectomy).

The medical record constructed by the first general practitioner was almost meaningless, with no indication that any examination of the lower bowel had occurred. Digital rectal examination is indicated in all patients who present with rectal bleeding. This maxim was established in the mid nineteenth century, and is still pertinent today. Furthermore, proctoscopic examination should be within the competence of any general practitioner.

Harry's 2007 general practitioner functioned merely as a referral clerk: no examination — simply consult a surgeon. This could not have been gratifying for the doctor in terms of job satisfaction. The failure to examine Harry properly meant that Harry was not seen by the surgeon until the following year. He denied Harry prompt and appropriate treatment, and reduced the chance of a favourable outcome.

It is worth noting that 10 years may elapse from the onset of a bowel polyp to development of carcinoma. The first general practitioner could have confidently detected the presence of the rectal polyp at the time of the first consultation, thus heightening the suspicion of development of cancer thereafter.

The surgeon discovered rectal cancer in 2008. He said that he would see Harry within a few weeks, and advised the referring practitioner accordingly. Harry did not understand the gravity of the situation. He believed that the surgical procedure of colonoscopy and biopsy had been curative.

If the surgeon had spoken to Harry at the end of the procedure while he was still affected by sedation, it is likely that Harry would not have understood the need for follow-up. Harry's partner stated that he did not attend the surgeon as requested for two reasons: firstly, he believed the surgical procedure was curative; secondly, he was not financially comfortable. If he had understood the gravity of the problem he would certainly have visited the surgeon. It is possible that Harry was reassured if it was the case that the rate of bleeding had slowed after the procedure; we do not know if that was the case.

It is tragic that neither the surgeon nor the referring general practitioner contacted Harry on receipt of the biopsy report to inform him of the need for urgent further care.

When Harry's partner requested that the histopathology report be faxed to the general practice clinic, the surgeon did not review the report. As a result, he offered no advice about follow-up. No one at the clinic appears to have reviewed the fax upon its receipt. It was simply added to Harry's record, and ignored thereafter.

The general practitioners provided the most superficial and unsatisfactory care. None of them reviewed the documentation of rectal cancer in Harry's record until he complained of altered bowel habit.

Another obvious example of less than competent practice was the prescription for varenicline without adequate advice. Fortunately this did not impact on Harry's welfare.

The obligation to provide continuing, comprehensive, whole patient care, the cornerstone of general practice, is difficult in a multidoctor practice. It is nonetheless a requirement that must be taken seriously, otherwise patients will suffer unnecessarily, as occurred in this case.

CLINICAL PRINCIPLES

This was a communication problem at all levels. Harry did not understand the importance of the findings at the colonoscopy, possibly because the conversation between him and the surgeon occurred when he was not fully alert.

The malignant potential of the large polyp, discovered at the time of the colonoscopy, was likely to have been understood by the surgeon at that time. He should have ensured that Harry and his partner understood the need for follow-up. It is unknown why the surgeon did not contact Harry within a few weeks of the procedure to ensure urgent review.

The latter general practice received the histopathology results and no one contacted Harry. It seems that the practitioner who saw Harry at that time either did not view the fax or for whatever reason did not contact Harry with the results.

Others in this practice did not appreciate the need to actively review histopathology results when they are received.

MISSED PERIOD

HISTORY

Lucy Simpson visited her general practitioner, Dr Tyson Harland, in 2005, as she was 10 days late for her menstrual period. Her obstetric history included a tubal pregnancy in 1994 that had been managed by salpingostomy, removal of the ectopic and tubal repair. One year later she had a normal vaginal delivery following an uncomplicated pregnancy. A spontaneous miscarriage followed two years after the normal delivery. In 2003 she had a nonviable pregnancy managed by dilation and curettage.

At the 2005 presentation Dr Harland performed an initial urine pregnancy test that was negative. He asked Lucy to return the following week for a repeat test. At the initial visit she had complained of urinary frequency, particularly in the morning. Dr Harland suggested that she might have a urinary tract infection, for which he prescribed antibiotics.

A week after the first visit Lucy felt nauseated and giddy with flu-like symptoms; she believed that she might have contracted the same virus as her son had suffered the previous week. She also stated that mosquitoes had bitten her earlier in the year and that she had experienced similar symptoms immediately thereafter.

Lucy told Dr Harland at this second consultation that she had commenced spotting. He stated that there was no point in performing a further pregnancy test, as this spotting indicated the commencement of a period. She also complained of dysuria. Dr Harland did not examine Lucy. He explained that she probably had thrush secondary to the antibiotic use; he prescribed clotrimazole cream for the possible fungal infection, and prochlorperazine for the nausea.

Three days later Lucy passed a large clot and other material vaginally. She felt nauseated and had cramping and lower abdominal pain. The locum general practitioner who visited her examined the material that she had passed, performed a thorough examination and diagnosed miscarriage. He suggested that she should have an ultrasound to ensure that the miscarriage had been complete. Lucy told the locum of her previous miscarriages and her previous ectopic pregnancy. He gave her a small supply of paracetamol with codeine, for analgesia.

Lucy saw Dr Harland the following day. He arranged a full blood count, blood group, quantitative βHCG and a pelvic ultrasound. The quantitative βHCG result of 1,404 IU/L (nonpregnant reference <10 IU/L) indicated pregnancy, gestation five to six weeks.

The ultrasound showed an empty uterus, normal endometrial thickness of 6.6 mm, right ovary 11.2 mm, left ovary of 9.9 mm, both within normal limits and a 2.0 cm possible old corpus luteum cyst. There was no adnexal mass or free fluid, and was no evidence of products of conception.

Ten days later Lucy contacted Dr Harland's rooms and was told that she was not pregnant (contrary to the βHCG evidence) and that continued spotting, abdominal pain and tenderness would pass in time.

Lucy decided to visit a different general practitioner. She was confident that she was not pregnant because of the assurance that she had been given. Her major reason for visiting the new doctor was to discuss sterilisation options. During the consultation she told the doctor that she had been unwell, had a recent bladder infection and was suffering from thrush. This doctor prescribed a different antibiotic for her supposed bladder infection. He performed a vaginal examination and a cervical smear, and commented that there was a small amount of blood on her cervix.

Two weeks later Lucy visited the second general practitioner again. He now had the results of the pathology tests and ultrasound performed five weeks previously. He informed Lucy that the pregnancy test had in fact been positive. No further advice was offered.

Two nights later Lucy awoke at 02:00 h with nausea and vomiting, generalised abdominal pain particularly on the right side, right shoulder tip pain, thirst, hot and cold sweats and dyspnoea. A locum visited her and arranged for her to be assessed at the regional obstetric hospital. When she arrived there she had a pulse rate of 84 bpm, respiratory rate of 26 breaths per minute, blood pressure of 120/70 mmHg and an axillary temperature of 38.0°C. She was tender at the right iliac fossa; the uterus appeared empty; there was bilateral tenderness in the fornices, and cervical excitation. Vaginal examination was difficult as Lucy was unable to lie flat. So she was examined in the lateral position. She required multiple injections of morphine.

βHCG remained elevated at 999 IU/L and she had a leucocytosis (white cell count 13.5×10^9/L, reference 4.3–10.8 $\times 10^9$/L). The CRP was normal at <5.0 mg/L (reference <5.0 mg/L), as was the haemoglobin concentration (122 g/L, reference 120–160 g/L). As she was unable to lie flat, only a limited pelvic ultrasound scan was possible. This showed a large amount of free fluid in the abdomen. The diagnosis was ectopic pregnancy; Lucy needed urgent surgery.

There was considerable delay before Lucy could be taken to the theatre, as there were several other patients requiring urgent care that morning. During the five hours from arrival at the hospital until she reached the theatre, Lucy's condition continued to deteriorate. Despite intravenous Haemaccel and normal saline, her systolic blood pressure dropped from 100 mmHg to 60 mmHg. Her haemoglobin fell to 45 g/L, for which she received four units of blood. Laparoscopy commenced two and a half hours following the ultrasound. Surgical findings were ruptured right tubal ectopic pregnancy and massive haemoperitoneum. Lucy stabilised after right salpingectomy.

Legal Issues

Lucy sought compensation for the consequences of delayed diagnosis and management of tubal pregnancy. The matter was settled at mediation.

Discussion

The nonpregnant βHCG level is <10 IU/L; levels of 999 IU/L and 1,404 IU/L indicated pregnancy. The empty uterus and elevated βHCG indicated ectopic pregnancy. Neither Dr Harland nor the second general practitioner understood this.

The principal diagnosis at the hospital was ectopic pregnancy. Although Lucy was febrile on arrival, and there was a mild leucocytosis, the CRP was normal, indicating that infection was not likely the primary problem.

The clinical findings at all stages of the progress of the illness indicated an ectopic pregnancy. Shoulder tip pain (due to subdiaphragmatic irritation) on presentation to the hospital was a classic symptom of intraperitoneal bleeding.

Clinical Principles

Ectopic pregnancy is a condition that still leads to maternal death. The possibility of such a diagnosis must be uppermost in the clinician's mind, particularly if a pregnancy is in any way unusual.

Dr Harland believed that a small amount of bleeding confirmed the beginning of a menstrual period, and was not due to an ectopic pregnancy. He was wrong.

All general practitioners may encounter pregnant women, not just those who practice obstetrics. All general practitioners must be familiar with diagnosing ectopic pregnancy, as this a potentially fatal condition for both mother and child.

There was considerable delay from the time Lucy arrived at the hospital until she could be surgically managed. That was certainly less than ideal but it was the reality of the situation.

Lucy's complications occurred early in the first trimester. In other circumstances, pregnant women who reside in regions where obstetric services are limited are encouraged to travel to a larger centre at 36 weeks gestation so that complications can be managed quickly and effectively.

Lucy had a real risk of losing her life due to delayed diagnosis and management of ectopic pregnancy. Better and earlier understanding of the clinical and investigation findings would likely have averted a potentially lethal situation.

AN OBSTETRIC ABNORMALITY

History

Pamela McNamara attended her usual doctor, Dr Megan Donoghue FRACGP, for a routine second trimester pregnancy ultrasound. Pamela's pregnancy was being managed on a shared care basis between her general practitioner and her obstetrician. Important findings from the ultrasound included cervical funnelling and a cervical length of 15 mm. The radiologist, who was concerned about the findings, telephoned Dr Donoghue to discuss the results. Dr Donoghue contacted Pamela four days later and asked her to visit the surgery to discuss the results. On her arrival Dr Donoghue did not offer to see her, rather Pamela was presented with a referral to her obstetrician and requested to make her own appointment.

Pamela was upset with Dr Donoghue's approach, as she was keen to be told the results of the ultrasound and to understand their implications. The next available appointment with the obstetrician was 11 days later. Pamela then opened the ultrasound report and following an internet search discovered the relevance of the findings. She contacted the obstetrician's surgery seeking to make an earlier appointment, either with that or a different obstetrician, only to discover that the doctor was unwilling to assist her prior to the appointment 11 days later. When Pamela suffered a miscarriage a week later she was grief stricken, as she believed that she had been badly managed.

Legal Issues

Pamela sought compensation from Dr Donoghue for the pain and suffering of the miscarriage and for the psychological impact of the loss of her baby.

She relied on the expert opinions of a general practitioner and obstetrician. The general practitioner maintained that it was inappropriate for Dr Donoghue to assume management of a pregnancy, even on a shared care basis, without having the expertise or willingness to recognise and act on abnormal examination results. It was unreasonable for Dr Donoghue to wait four days after the radiologist's warning about the ultrasound results before doing anything about it. And then when she acted on the results she did nothing but write a referral to the obstetrician. The general practitioner expert was highly critical of this response.

An obstetric expert was of the view that earlier referral and treatment may have avoided the miscarriage.

It is yet to be seen whether Dr Donoghue's lawyers will identify a general practitioner prepared to support her conduct.

The case is ongoing.

Discussion

The radiologist was sufficiently concerned with the ultrasound findings that he contacted Dr Donoghue directly. Radiologists do not usually phone referrers to discuss benign results. It was appropriate practice for the radiologist to phone Dr Donoghue if he was concerned about abnormal findings, and it indicated that urgent management was required. Dr Donoghue did not arrange such urgent consultant obstetric review, thus abrogating her responsibility of providing adequate patient care. There was an unreasonable mismatch between her response and that of the radiologist.

It is well understood in obstetric practice that patients with an ultrasonographic cervical length ≤15 mm have ~50% risk of early spontaneous preterm delivery: it is difficult to understand the mindset of Dr Donoghue. Whether she was distracted by other matters is unclear. She had a shared care arrangement with the local obstetrician and, even if she was unaware of the implications of a shortened cervix, she must have known that the radiologist would not have contacted her directly if he had not been concerned. The correct response was to contact the obstetrician directly to discuss the matter and to obtain guidance. Pamela should not have been left in the dark or reliant on Google to advance her own interests.

It is also noted that, on receipt of the call from the radiologist about an urgent matter, Dr Donoghue waited for four days before contacting Pamela. Even then, Dr Donoghue declined to see Pamela to discuss the matter. She appeared disinterested in Pamela's welfare.

Clinical Principles

The international literature describing the role of the general practitioner emphasises the notion of being the patient's advocate. Dr Donoghue was a fellow of The Royal Australian College of General Practitioners. She knows that this fellowship carries with it the responsibility to provide continuing, comprehensive, whole patient care.

Dr Donoghue was neither Pamela's advocate nor provided her with continuing or comprehensive care.

While patients must be encouraged to take responsibility for their own health, this does not mean that the fundamental role of primary health care providers like general practitioners can be diluted.

PLACENTA PERCRETA

HISTORY

Simone and Rod Beall were married in 2007. In 2008 Simone delivered their first child, Kate, by emergency caesarean section following a diagnosis of cord prolapse. Unfortunately, Kate suffered hypoxic-ischaemic brain damage and was subsequently diagnosed with cerebral palsy. One year later, in 2009, Simone again fell pregnant. She and Rod were excited, but understandably anxious about the outcome of the pregnancy. They attended antenatal consultations together, and were relieved when Simone's general practitioner referred her to the maternal fetal medicine (MFM) unit at a Melbourne metropolitan hospital for management of the pregnancy and delivery. At the time of the second pregnancy, Simone and Rod were both 27 years of age. Both had graduated with a law degree and were working in large firms in Melbourne. Simone had found it difficult to return to work after Kate's birth because of the constant need for care. She had reduced her working hours to a part-time capacity and relied on her family for significant support.

Simone and Rod first attended the MFM unit at the hospital on 23 May 2009 at 19 weeks gestation. An ultrasound was performed, which revealed a grade 4 placenta praevia (low lying placenta) and at least a placenta accreta (placenta growing too deeply into the uterine wall). As a result of the previous caesarean section delivery, the placenta had become adherent to the anterior wall of the uterus with the vessels extending into and possibly through the uterus into the wall of the bladder (placenta percreta). There was a very thin anterior uterine wall suggesting almost complete invasion of the placental tissue through the wall (placenta increta or percreta).

Simone attended the MFM unit on seven occasions. On each occasion, she was examined by Dr Rupert Franks, the staff specialist in obstetrics and gynaecology and a MFM subspecialist, as well as Dr Jane Dunn, the obstetrics and gynaecology registrar. On each occasion, the placenta was noted on ultrasound examination, including Doppler flow studies, to be into or through the uterine wall, but recorded in the notes as only being a placenta accreta and a placenta praevia grade 4.

Because of the placenta accreta and the proximity to the bladder, Simone and Rod were advised that there was a risk of significant bleeding and the need for a blood transfusion, hysterectomy or even a cystectomy. Simone was advised by both Dr Franks and Dr Dunn to undergo an elective caesarean section delivery, the incision being made through the same incision used for Kate's delivery (a Pfannenstiel incision), with a subsequent incision into the lower uterine segment of the uterus where the previous entry into the uterus had been achieved. Acting on the advice of Doctors Franks and Dunn, Simone consented to the proposed operation. Rod agreed.

On 17 October 2009, Simone was admitted to the hospital for elective caesarean section delivery. At 13:30 h on 18 October 2008, Simone and Rod's second child, Robert, was delivered by a lower segment caesarean section.

Dr Franks permitted Dr Dunn to be the lead surgeon for the operation. Under his supervision, Dr Dunn reflected the bladder away from the anterior surface of the uterus. This was difficult because the bladder wall appeared to be adherent to the lower uterus. Dr Dunn could not completely reflect the bladder from the uterine wall. Despite this, she then opened the uterus using the prior lower segment incision. Dr Dunn tentatively expanded the initial incision and was met by placental tissue. The placental tissue bled heavily. Once Robert was delivered, the placental tissue could only be removed piecemeal. It was deeply adherent to the wall of the uterus. When touched, it bled profusely. Simone suffered a torrential haemorrhage. She was administered numerous blood transfusions and intravenous fluid. She developed disseminated intravascular coagulation (DIC). Dr Dunn, with Dr Franks' concurrence, opted for a subtotal hysterectomy, which failed to stem the bleeding. Packs were pushed into the uterus and pelvis to no avail. They sought the assistance of other surgeons, including a urologist. He was not able to avert the catastrophe. Simone suffered a cardiac arrest from the hypovolaemic shock and died at the age of 27, leaving behind a husband, an infant daughter with cerebral palsy and a healthy newborn baby boy.

Legal Issues

Rod commenced proceedings for nervous shock and a dependency claim against the hospital, given that Simone was treated as a public patient and that Doctors Franks and Dunn were employees of the hospital.

There was also an inquest into Simone's death. The coroner found that the death could not have been avoided.

Rod, acting on legal advice and expert opinion, disagreed with the coroner's findings, and gave instructions to commence civil proceedings.

Batteries of experts were relied on by both sides, including obstetricians, gynaecological oncologists, interventional radiologists and MFM specialists. Rod argued that his wife's death could have been avoided by a number of simple, sensible steps.

First, there should have been careful matching of the experience and expertise required for the operation and the grave risks associated with the procedure. Dr Franks was a recent appointment as a staff specialist in obstetrics and gynaecology and a subspecialist in MFM. He had very little experience in cases of placenta increta or percreta. He had never performed such complex, risky surgery. Dr Dunn was a registrar. She had never come across such a case. Neither of them had experience in difficult pelvic dissections, which are usually performed by gynaecological oncologists. While Doctors Franks and Dunn had the experience to perform a caesarean section and to evaluate patients attending the MFM unit of the hospital, they were underqualified to perform the surgery required for delivery of Simone's child.

The experts relied on by the plaintiff also suggested there should have been better planning for the operation. An interventional radiologist and gynaecological oncologist or experienced gynaecologist ought to have been brought into the team to advise. Given that the antenatal ultrasounds suggested possible placenta praevia percreta, it could reasonably be anticipated that there would be terrible bleeding in the absence of preventative steps. It was unsafe to assume Simone had placenta accreta rather than a more invasive form of the problem. Preoperative embolisation of key arteries by an interventional radiologist would have minimised the risk of fatal haemorrhage. In addition, a gynaecological oncologist was more likely to be able to perform difficult dissections if the operation proved hazardous, including accessing and tying off arteries at the pelvic sidewalls.

Rod also alleged that he and his wife were never informed of the risk of death associated with the operation and hence how serious it was. They were never given the opportunity to request more experienced surgeons. They assumed that Doctors Franks and Dunn had the necessary experience.

The doctors' lack of experience was also manifest by a number of intraoperative decisions they made. It was imprudent to use a Pfannenstiel incision in the lower abdomen rather than a vertical abdominal incision, which would have enabled the surgeon to have greater access to the abdominal cavity in the event of bleeding. In addition, the decision to cut through the uterus at the site of the previous scar made damage to the placenta almost inevitable. Dr Dunn could not reflect the bladder from the anterior uterine wall because it was densely adherent to it. This ought to have suggested invasion of the placenta through the wall into the bladder as suggested on antenatal ultrasounds. The error in cutting through the previous uterine scar was compounded by the decision to remove the placenta piecemeal when the only foreseeable outcome would be torrential haemorrhage. Once the bleeding appeared uncontrollable, the proper salvage operation was a total hysterectomy rather than a sub-total hysterectomy. Critical time was lost with tying up arteries, which would have been more effectively dealt with by a gynaecological oncologist.

The case settled at mediation.

Discussion

This case represents an extreme example of doctors not appreciating the limits of their clinical acumen. Simone and Rod Beall thought they had been referred to the very best care for Simone's second pregnancy. They understood that placenta praevia accreta was a serious condition and that, following delivery, a hysterectomy or cystectomy may be necessary. They assumed the expertise and experience of Doctors Franks and Dunn. They were not given any information about their experience in dealing with such a complex problem as placenta praevia accreta. They were not told of the risk of death. Further, they were not told about the probability of the growth of the placenta through the wall of the bladder to be complete so that in truth Simone had a placenta praevia percreta rather than accreta.

It is frequently the case that a disgruntled patient suffering a complication from surgery complains that he or she was not told that the operation would be performed by a trainee rather than the consultant. These complaints are rarely of any moment. The registrar is usually supervised adequately. It is impossible to train doctors to become specialist surgeons if they do not gain experience first-hand in the public hospital system. This case is not about an operation being performed by a registrar rather than the consultant. This is a case where the degree of complexity of the surgery was above the competence of *both* the consultant and the registrar.

What should have happened was that more experienced gynaecological surgeons or gynaecological oncologists should have been brought into the team to advise and perform the surgery. Proper preparation involving a senior anaesthetist, gynaecological oncologist and interventional radiologist would have maximised the chances of survival. The choices made by Doctors Franks and Dunn in collaboration with each other were decisions that failed to reflect their accumulated clinical judgment. It was like being in an echo chamber, repeatedly hearing their own views; finally being convinced that their choices were correct. Dr Franks ought to have recognised that he was outside a safe zone of practice. There was no evidence about why he chose to go it alone with his registrar, but it was a decision that may have contributed to Simone's death. Perhaps Dr Franks found it difficult to communicate to more senior specialists given his recent appointment as a staff specialist. It may have been an example of the authority gradient in operation. Dr Dunn certainly did not challenge Dr Franks' opinions. It is possible that the two lacked insight or had distorted insight into their own abilities.

Clinical Principles

The practice of medicine depends upon effective communication. Communication occurs between doctors and patients, doctors and nurses, and between professional colleagues. To be able to communicate effectively, it is first necessary to appreciate that one has a need to communicate a particular issue. Many years ago, a paternalistic approach to medicine often meant that patients were largely kept in the dark about risks associated with proposed treatment. The adage "doctor knows best" meant that patients rarely questioned their doctors.

Multidisciplinary teams have been established in most hospitals to ensure that the opinions of specialists across a range of disciplines are heard to enable the best decision to be made in the interests of a patient. The lack of such a collaborative approach by Doctors Franks and Dunn meant that Simone and Rod did not receive valuable input from specialists who could have provided guidance to the operating surgeons to take steps that may have avoided the tragedy. Proper education about the need to communicate and collaborate with colleagues must continue.

PELVIC ORGAN PROLAPSE

History

In early 2006, at the age of 44, Christine Talbot first experienced the symptoms of vaginal prolapse. She had minor dyspareunia (discomfort with sexual intercourse) and a feeling of a bulge at the introitus, particularly at the end of the day. She had delivered three children vaginally between 1987 and 1997. She was happily married and otherwise healthy.

As a result of the vaginal prolapse, her general practitioner referred Christine to Dr Gary Anderson, the obstetrician and gynaecologist who had delivered her children.

Christine consulted Dr Anderson on 26 April 2007. He elicited the history of the recent onset of a vaginal bulge and discomfort with intercourse. Christine did not report any urinary or bowel symptoms. On examination, Dr Anderson found an anterior vaginal prolapse (cystocoele), but no apical or posterior prolapse (rectocoele). During a Valsalva manoeuvre, the anterior wall of the vagina descended about 1 cm below the hymenal ring.

After his examination, Dr Anderson advised Christine that she needed to have surgery to repair her pelvic organ prolapse (POP). He advised that she needed an anterior repair to hold up her bladder. While the bowel had not yet prolapsed, he said he would check whether there was any weakening in the posterior compartment at the time of the operation. If it was weakened, then he recommended posterior repair as well. He also recommended that she undergo a vaginal hysterectomy at the same time. Rather than a traditional native repair (colporrhaphy), Dr Anderson suggested that her prolapse surgery be augmented with polypropylene mesh using a transvaginal mesh kit called GYNECARE PROLIFT®.

The device was a pelvic floor repair system manufactured by Ethicon Sàrl and distributed in Australia by Johnson & Johnson Pty Ltd. It was made from knitted filaments of nonabsorbable extruded polypropylene and inserted transvaginally with a set of special instruments. It was available for use between 2005 and 2013.

Dr Anderson explained the proposed procedure to Christine. He said the mesh sheets would be inserted between the posterior wall of the bladder and the anterior wall of the vagina. If there were posterior prolapse on examination under anaesthesia, then he would insert a sheet of mesh between the posterior vaginal wall and the anterior wall of the rectum. He indicated to Christine that, by using the mesh, she would be back at work sooner and that the repair would be long-lasting when compared with nonmesh surgery. This was preferable to traditional POP repair without mesh, which had a tendency to recur.

He said that the reason mesh was being used was because conventional surgery had a high failure rate. If there is failure, a patient will usually have more operations. This can lead to narrowing, shortening and scarring of the vagina, and can make sexual intercourse difficult or impossible. He went on to say that, unlike conventional surgery, mesh surgery takes place in the natural space between the vagina and the bladder, so the vagina does not need to be shortened or trimmed.

He said that he had performed a significant number of PROLIFT® operations and had been trained in the technique. Finally, he advised her that the PROLIFT® mesh surgery had been performed overseas over the previous five years and was very successful. He said it was the best option for her.

After the discussion, Dr Anderson provided Christine with a variety of documents and a consent form to sign. Those documents included a pamphlet on POP repair using PROLIFT® written by Ethicon Sàrl, a pamphlet entitled "Surgical Treatment of Pelvic Organ Prolapse" published by the Royal Australian and New Zealand College of Obstetricians and Gynaecologists (RANZCOG), and a long-form consent document authored by Dr Anderson, which set out some of the uncommon risks associated with mesh surgery. This document stated that several of his patients had experienced erosion of the mesh, but that it was easy to treat if it occurred.

The Ethicon brochure described PROLIFT® as "revolutionary". It also claimed that surgery with mesh was different from other surgical alternatives, because it could be completed in less than half the time of traditional surgery, and patients could experience less pain, have a quicker recovery and go home the next day. It also said that it allowed for the restoration of sexual function. There was a small risk of mesh eroding into the vagina.

The RANZCOG pamphlet contained the following in the section on vaginal mesh procedures:

> *In recent years, new techniques have been developed that use very small incisions around the vagina and anus to insert supporting mesh under the vaginal vault. Large pieces of mesh can be inserted in a similar manner to provide support to the vaginal walls. These procedures are minimally invasive, but long-term data is still being compiled on the effectiveness and complication rate. These procedures are generally indicated for patients with recurrent prolapse.*

Under the section concerning possible complications of surgery, the following was written:

> *Complications of the mesh affect about one in 10 to 20 women, such as inflammation near the mesh, failure of tissues to heal around the mesh, or mesh rejection. If this complication is severe, the mesh may need to be removed. Rarely, the mesh can erode into other organs such as the bowel or bladder and cause pain during intercourse.*

Based upon Dr Anderson's advice, both oral and written, Christine agreed to undergo POP repair surgery with PROLIFT®. She had the impression that native tissue repair was essentially obsolete, and that POP surgery with mesh was the only sensible option for her. She also was under the impression that POP repair surgery with PROLIFT® was a tried and tested method. Although the risk of mesh erosion was mentioned, Christine thought that it was a rare occurrence, and that if it materialised, it was easy to treat.

In August 2006, Dr Anderson operated on Christine. On examination under anaesthesia, Dr Anderson found a mild rectocoele. In consequence, he performed both an anterior and a posterior mesh repair using PROLIFT® together with a vaginal hysterectomy.

Christine had no immediate problems after the surgery. Two months later, however, Dr Anderson reoperated on Christine because she had developed mesh erosion through the anterior vaginal wall. He excised a 1-cm piece of exposed mesh. About one year later Christine underwent further surgery to remove mesh eroding into her vagina and bladder wall. By 2008, Christine also had mesh erosion in the posterior compartment. She underwent further surgery for mesh-related complications; the mesh had eroded into the posterior vaginal wall and into her rectum.

No further surgery was considered because removal of the mesh around the rectum and bladder was considered too hazardous. As a result, Christine is left with intractable pelvic pain, dyspareunia and an adjustment disorder with depression. She also has vaginal narrowing and alteration in her urinary and evacuatory function.

While she had some discomfort with sexual intercourse prior to her surgery, it was nothing like the pain she now experiences. In addition, her husband reported pain with intercourse, caused by penile lacerations due to the mesh eroding through the vaginal wall. Christine's chronic pain and dyspareunia has placed significant strains on her marital relationship.

Legal Issues

In 2010, Christine commenced proceedings in negligence against Dr Anderson for recommending and performing vaginal POP repair surgery with PROLIFT®. The essence of her case was that he failed to inform her adequately of the risk of mesh erosion associated with the use of PROLIFT®, and that he failed to give her accurate advice about the risks and benefits of POP repair surgery with mesh compared with POP repair surgery without mesh.

She specifically alleged that he misrepresented the safety and efficacy of POP repair with PROLIFT®. He portrayed a device of proven safety and effectiveness when, in fact, there were no reliable studies establishing that it was more effective and safer than conventional non-mesh POP repair.

Christine alleged that, if she had been properly advised about the absence of reliable evidence in relation to the safety and efficacy of PROLIFT®, the magnitude of the risks of mesh erosion, chronic pain and dyspareunia together with the potential seriousness of those risks if they eventuated (unable to be remedied because it was too hazardous to remove all of the mesh), she would never have consented to the operation, but would have instead undergone a native tissue repair.

The proceedings were hard fought because Dr Anderson sought to implicate the manufacturer and distributor of the product, which were respondents in a class action. The experts qualified by Christine were firmly of the view that she should have been told that POP repair with PROLIFT® was associated with significant risks of mesh erosion, chronic pain and dyspareunia, which were not easy to treat. They also considered that the evidence supporting the device's efficacy was limited.

The device was wanting altogether for posterior repairs, and had only been demonstrated in short-term studies in relation to anatomic rather than subjective cure. The experts retained by Dr Anderson pointed to the fact that PROLIFT® had been registered for use by the Therapeutic Goods Administration (TGA) as a Class II medical device, and therefore Dr Anderson was justified in using it. As there was no dispute that POP surgery was indicated, the use of an available device was reasonable in the circumstances. They thought his warnings were adequate.

The case settled at mediation.

Discussion

This case highlights the dangers of using new technology and the need to keep abreast of the literature in relation to the benefits and risks of that technology. While innovation is an important aspect of medical science and patient health, there must be limits on the uptake of new technology, and attention to the risks and benefits of that technology before rejecting what was previously thought to be the gold standard treatment in a particular area.

If accepted at trial, Christine's version of events was that she was never told that the long-term safety and efficacy of the mesh implants had been established. She also alleged that she was never told that posterior repair with PROLIFT® had never been demonstrated as being as efficacious or effective as native tissue repair.

While anterior repair with mesh had been shown to have better or equivalent anatomical cure as native tissue repair, it came with an increased incidence of complications and mesh-specific complications in the form of erosions and extrusion into adjacent organs resulting in chronic pain or chronic dyspareunia. Christine alleged that she was never told about the quality of the evidence available to establish the safety and efficacy of the implants. If she had known that it was, in essence, experimental, she would not have consented to the procedure. While the RANZCOG pamphlet referred to the risk of erosion and that long-term data were still being compiled, Dr Anderson's message to her was potentially contradictory and tended to undermine the cautious message in the pamphlet.

Clinical Principles

The context in which the information was provided to Christine was one of trust (Dr Anderson had delivered her children), and one where he must have known that she would follow any advice he gave. From Dr Anderson's perspective, the information was given in circumstances where he had effectively abandoned traditional prolapse surgery and only performed mesh repair surgery. This scenario meant that he was unlikely to give unbiased recommendations to the patient.

Class II medical devices can be registered with the Therapeutic Goods Administration without the manufacturer or distributor proving safety through a randomised clinical trial. The situation is more stringent for pharmaceuticals. Medical practitioners are unlikely to know this. While a specialist has a duty to keep abreast of the scientific literature relevant to the treatment options he or she may use, that duty falls short of being aware of all the literature on a particular topic. Some medical practitioners may not read the scientific literature on biomaterials or in vitro testing of new devices, which may nonetheless be relevant to the treatment they recommend to patients.

For these reasons, a doctor must approach new technology with some caution, especially if it is an implantable device where a learning curve is likely to exist. As a general rule, the enthusiastic and uncritical adoption of new technology is unlikely to be in the interest of patients.

A MESH BY ANY OTHER NAME

History

Following the birth of her fourth child, Sue Massey gradually noticed a bulge just outside the entry to her vagina. It was most apparent at the end of the day or after physical activity. It returned readily back into the vagina at night. The bulge was associated with a mild backache. Sue also noticed urinary frequency, urgency and nocturia. Very occasionally, she leaked urine with exertion or when coughing, laughing or sneezing. She had no problems with her bowels.

Sue was not planning to have any more children and thought it was time to treat the bulge. She consulted her general practitioner, Dr Wendy Horsley. Dr Horsley diagnosed Sue as having vaginal prolapse and recommended referral to a gynaecologist. Dr Horsley mentioned that there were new methods of treating vaginal prolapse, including with the use of mesh to support the vaginal walls. Sue was unsure about the use of mesh and wanted to research the topic before being referred to a gynaecologist.

After the consultation, Sue searched the internet for information about the treatment of pelvic organ prolapse (POP) and the use of vaginal mesh. She read of women suffering serious complications from the use of vaginal mesh, including chronic pain, vaginal erosions and difficulty removing the mesh if complications developed. Sue formed the strong view that she did not want to have treatment with polypropylene mesh. In the process of searching the internet, Sue came across a website for Professor Gavin Mulcahy. The website indicated that Professor Mulcahy was an advocate against the use of polypropylene mesh in the repair of POP. He held himself out as being a world-renowned gynaecological surgeon specialising in pelvic floor reconstruction. He also advertised himself as a fellow of multiple local and international colleges. Because of Professor Mulcahy's stand against mesh and his apparent expertise and experience in POP repair, Sue contacted Dr Horsley for a referral to see Professor Mulcahy.

On 21 October 2013, at the age of 40, Sue consulted Professor Mulcahy. He had an excellent bedside manner. His voice was mellifluous. He seemed charming, compassionate and knowledgeable. He examined Sue and took a history. He also asked her to complete a questionnaire covering issues such as urinary function, bowel function, sexual function and the vaginal bulge. He diagnosed Sue as suffering from an exteriorising cystocoele, rectocoele and urge incontinence. He recommended a number of investigations, including a transperineal ultrasound, urodynamic studies and an MRI scan of the pelvic floor (static and dynamic), together with a fluoroscopic proctogram.

Professor Mulcahy performed the transperineal ultrasound himself. He also performed a 3D/4D ultrasound. In his opinion, the scans demonstrated a large diffuse cystocoele and a moderate-sized rectocoele. He then performed urodynamic studies. These demonstrated a small residual volume of urine, but no other abnormality. There was no detrusor overactivity or genuine stress urinary incontinence (SUI). The MRI scan was performed by a radiologist. The radiologist reported some drooping of the lower third of the vagina, but no significant cystocoele and a small, borderline, rectocoele. There was no evidence of a tear to any of the supporting structures of the urethra or vagina or to the anal sphincter complex. The proctogram demonstrated a small rectocoele, which was not apparent at rest.

On 30 November 2013, Sue returned to discuss the findings of the investigations with Professor Mulcahy. Professor Mulcahy recommended an anterior and posterior repair to treat the cystocoele and rectocoele. He informed Sue that he would use a biological graft to strengthen the repair but would not be using any polypropylene mesh. He advised her that he had obtained good, anatomic results with the use of a biological graft. Based upon the advice and information provided to her, Sue consented to the surgery.

On 16 December 2013, Professor Mulcahy operated on Sue at a private hospital. Professor Mulcahy purportedly found at operation a stage III cystourethrocoele, a left paravaginal defect, a stage III rectocoele, a deficiency in the left uterosacral ligament and moderate stress incontinence. He went on to perform what he called a vaginal sacrocolpopexy, an anterior and posterior repair and mid-urethral sling placement using the Tissue Fixation System (TFS). TFS was a system for the surgical treatment of POP and SUI that involved the insertion of multiple nonabsorbable, polypropylene, pronged anchors within the pelvis through which nonabsorbable, polypropylene mesh tapes were threaded and secured.

Professor Mulcahy inserted five TFS devices into Sue's pelvis. His notes recorded that the first TFS tape and anchor was used to stabilise the bladder base. The second TFS tape and anchor was advanced along the uterosacral ligament tunnel to the sacral hollow. A third TFS tape and anchor was placed in the pararectal tunnel and a fourth TFS tape and anchor was inserted underneath the urethra. A tape and anchor was also inserted through the perineal body.

Following the operation, Sue immediately developed urinary retention. Professor Mulcahy cut the mid-urethral tape. Sue then developed severe pelvic, vaginal, perineal, buttock and lower back pain. She sought an explanation from Professor Mulcahy. It was at this time that Professor Mulcahy told her that he had inserted a number of TFS tapes and anchors in her pelvis. He told her they were made from polypropylene but assured her that the amount of polypropylene mesh in the TFS was minimal and nothing like the amount of polypropylene used in the transvaginal mesh he abhorred. Nonetheless, Sue was aghast at the news. She could not believe that Professor

Mulcahy had not told her about the use of polypropylene. She confronted him about it.

According to Professor Mulcahy, he said that he had mentioned the use of the TFS prior to the operation and had informed Dr Horsley to that effect. A letter to Dr Horsley confirmed that TFS had been mentioned. He also said that TFS was mentioned on the consent form Sue had signed. Sue said she thought that was the biological graft he had mentioned. He replied that he had found that TFS gave better results and thus had decided to use it.

Sue subsequently developed vaginal exposure of one of the tapes. Professor Mulcahy advised her to have the tape removed and attempted to do so during two operations. Sue's pain persisted. She developed dyspareunia and eventually apareunia because of the intense pain associated with sexual intercourse. She also had urge incontinence and defaecatory obstruction. She was diagnosed with a chronic pain syndrome which was intractable and unable to be alleviated by any means. Sue's relationship with her husband deteriorated. She was unable to perform many of the domestic and child-rearing tasks she had performed before. She was unable to participate in many of the physical activities and sports she had engaged in before the operation. She was unable to work. The surgery dramatically altered her life.

Legal Issues

Sue engaged lawyers to investigate suing Professor Mulcahy in negligence and also complained to the Health Care Complaints Commission (HCCC) about Professor Mulcahy's conduct. The case involved questions about the provision of information and representations made by Professor Mulcahy, the adequacy of the consent process, whether the operation was properly indicated and performed in a competent manner, and whether the TFS system was a valid, safe and efficacious form of POP repair surgery or surgery for SUI.

Sue's lawyers obtained opinions from three urogynaecologists, a gynaecologist, a gynaecologist specialising in pain management and a psychiatrist. All of the gynaecologists were of the opinion that the TFS had resulted in a chronic pain syndrome, which affected urinary, bowel and sexual function. There had also been a recurrence of Sue's POP. This could not be repaired because of the presence of the TFS tape and anchors, which could not be removed safely. There was also a consensus in relation to the need for the surgery performed by Professor Mulcahy. As Sue did not have urodynamically-proven SUI, there was no need to insert a mid-urethral tape.

Secondly, there was no reason to perform a posterior repair because the rectocoele was either very small or borderline and, more importantly, was not causing any bowel symptoms. They maintained that there was a dearth of evidence supporting the use of TFS through the perineal body. They agreed, however, that it was reasonable to recommend and perform an anterior repair, but not with any form of mesh given that it was a primary repair and Sue did not wish to have any polypropylene inserted inside her.

They were all critical of the consent process and the information provided to Sue about whether TFS had proven safety and efficacy, and the risks and complications associated with the use of transvaginal polypropylene products. It was misleading to distinguish TFS from other polypropylene mesh kits with known complications. There had been numerous publications by the Royal Australian and New Zealand College of Obstetricians and Gynaecologists (RANZCOG) as well as the United States Food and Drug Administration (FDA). Sue should have been provided information contained in those guidelines.

Finally, when complications ensued, Professor Mulcahy should have referred her to a skilled urogynaecologist. He had only started deploying TFS shortly before Sue's surgery and had had limited training in its use.

Professor Mulcahy relied on the opinion of two gynaecologists. They maintained that TFS had been registered for use by the Therapeutic Goods Administration and was on the Australian Register of Therapeutic Goods (ARTG). Accordingly, it was reasonable for a gynaecologist to use the registered device for its intended purpose. They also maintained that the TFS had been shown to be safe and efficacious, including its use through the perineal body. They considered anterior and posterior repairs were reasonably indicated and, as Sue had some symptoms of SUI, the insertion of a suburethral tape was also indicated. Sue's experts argued that TFS had not been subjected to any long-term clinical studies to evaluate its safety and efficacy in the surgical treatment of POP, SUI or when passed through the perineal body. TFS has subsequently been taken off the ARTG.

There was a dispute about the adequacy of the information provided to Sue by Professor Mulcahy, but this contest depended on whose version of events one accepted as being true. The gynaecologists supporting Professor Mulcahy's conduct effectively asserted that because Professor Mulcahy had a wealth of experience and knowledge in POP surgery and it was his usual practice to discuss the information about proposed surgery in a detailed way, it was unlikely he failed to advise Sue of all material risks or issues. At the time of the surgery, the FDA had promulgated statements in October 2008 and July 2011 about the use of transvaginal mesh. The RANZCOG had published guidelines on the use of transvaginal mesh in March 2013. There were Cochrane reviews about the safety and efficacy of the use of transvaginal mesh for the treatment of POP. Professor Mulcahy's experts said they expected he was across this information. Neither went as far as saying that Professor Mulcahy provided this information to Sue. This was unsurprising as Professor Mulcahy's clinical notes and records were silent in relation to the issue of warnings, risks and alternative treatment options. This was contrary to the requirements of the Health Practitioner Regulation (NSW) 2012, which specifically mandates that the information and advice given to a patient is to be recorded.

From 15 September 2011, Professor Mulcahy had conditions placed on his practising certificate. Professor Mulcahy was not permitted to perform antiincontinence surgery without urodynamic studies and was not permitted to perform 3D/4D ultrasound investigations without the benefit of an independent expert review. While he performed urodynamic studies, he ignored them when he chose to insert a suburethral tape. The urodynamic studies failed to find SUI. In addition, he performed the ultrasound contrary to the restrictions on his practice.

Despite the service of expert reports on his behalf, it was difficult to ascertain Professor Mulcahy's reasons for using a largely untried device for the primary treatment of POP or to insert a suburethral tape when Sue did not have SUI. It was also difficult to comprehend how he believed it was appropriate to use polypropylene products when he had categorically informed the general public on his website and specifically to Sue that he did not use such products and was vehemently opposed to their use.

Sue's civil proceedings were settled after mediation.

The HCCC prosecuted a claim against Professor Mulcahy in the NSW Civil and Administrative Tribunal (NCAT) in relation to his management of a number of women. NCAT published its decision in 2018. Professor Mulcahy ceased practice before the reasons were published. It found that Professor Mulcahy failed to implement individualised care plans to his patients' detriment, while his clinical errors of judgment were made often and without appropriate warnings and information to patients. It found that he failed to seek a referral or obtain a second opinion before surgery or to conduct further investigations. He failed to follow the RANZCOG guidelines about the information to be provided to patients about mesh and he failed to keep adequate records. He also breached his conditions of registration.

NCAT made orders that would have cancelled Professor Mulcahy's registration (if he had not already ceased practice) and disqualified him from being registered for five years.

Discussion

This case highlights the importance of full and frank disclosure about the safety and efficacy of new products or surgical techniques together with information about the individual practitioner's experience with their use. A good bedside manner is no substitute for competent practice. It is no substitute for proper informed consent. Medical practitioners should be alive to the power imbalance intrinsic to the doctor–patient relationship. The majority of patients are unlikely to be aware when they are being misled. A layperson is not going to appreciate nuances in a proposed treatment. Practitioners who do not appreciate the power imbalance or exploit it for their own benefit should not be practising medicine.

The case also highlights the vexed question as to whether conditions placed on a doctor's right to practice should be available to the public or should be part of the information disclosed to a patient. If conditions are disclosed to patients, then there may be a natural hesitancy in undergoing treatment by that doctor compared with a doctor of the same speciality without any practice restrictions. A doctor's capacity to earn income may be compromised. On the other hand, if a patient is unaware of the restrictions, they may not appreciate that the doctor is straying outside of the areas in which he is entitled to give treatment. Patient safety should be the paramount determinant.

In addition, the case again highlights the problems associated with the introduction of new medical devices or technologies. The assumption that a product has been properly tested and evaluated because it is on the ARTG is not always correct. But the majority of medical practitioners probably think that this assumption is reasonable. Medical practitioners require education about what it means for a product to be on the ARTG. It does not necessarily mean their safety and efficacy have been adequately assessed.

In any event, a doctor owes patients a duty to keep reasonably up-to-date with the scientific knowledge relevant to the treatment he or she recommends and provides to patients. The fact that a device may be listed on the ARTG should not absolve a practitioner from keeping abreast of the literature relevant to his area of practice.

The case highlights the need to pay attention to the details of studies to assess whether they are relevant to a particular patient's circumstances. Further education may be necessary in epidemiology to enable medical practitioners to evaluate scientific papers more critically.

Clinical Principles

It is important for a medical practitioner to understand the limits of his or her skills and knowledge. While it is perfectly reasonable to embark upon the use of new technologies, adequate training and reading ought to occur first. A lack of experience needs to be discussed with a patient. No patient wants to feel as if he or she is a guinea pig. They need to be reassured. Avoidance of the issue is inappropriate, but a doctor needs to have the confidence to be able tackle the issue.

There is also nothing wrong with providing information about one's training, experience and particular expertise on a website or by other means. Indeed, such information is beneficial to patients when deciding what to do. This, however, should not be a licence to behave as a salesperson or to provide inaccurate information to lure patients to one's practice. The power imbalance in the doctor–patient relationship should not be exploited.

FAILED HIP REPLACEMENT

History

On 10 October 2015, Jake Toohey underwent a right total hip replacement at a private hospital. His orthopaedic surgeon was Dr Lewis Shadbolt. Dr Shadbolt specialised in hip and knee replacement surgery. Jake had been a rugby league player. At the age of 45, his knees and hips were starting to give him pain with his right hip being the worst. He had been diagnosed with osteoarthritis of the hip. It was painful and his range of movement was significantly restricted.

The operation went well. Dr Shadbolt performed the operation using a ceramic implant. There were no immediate problems.

After his recovery in the initial few days, Dr Shadbolt referred Jake for inpatient rehabilitation under the care of rehabilitation physician, Dr Mark Carey. Dr Carey not only prescribed physiotherapy and hydrotherapy, but also undertook to look at the wound from time to time.

One week later, as he was undergoing physiotherapy in the rehabilitation ward, Jake noticed that his wound was oozing and leaking a bloody, red fluid.

Nursing staff changed the bandages, which were soaked, and replaced them. He was advised to slow down with physiotherapy and hydrotherapy. Dr Shadbolt reviewed the wound and ordered a pressure dressing. There was never any evidence of cellulitis.

By 20 October 2015, the wound was still leaking. Jake felt slightly nauseous and on the previous day felt as though he had a fever.

On 21 October 2015, Dr Shadbolt ordered a swab to be taken of the wound for culture and sensitivity, and prescribed oral antibiotics (Keflex) for five days. Dr Shadbolt recorded in the notes that the wound needed to be reviewed on 22 October 2015.

The wound swab grew methicillin-sensitive Staphylococcus aureus (MSSA). The forms recording the results were sent by the pathology laboratory to the rehabilitation ward on 23 October 2015. The results were also disseminated electronically to Dr Carey and the rehabilitation ward.

From 23 October 2015, Dr Shadbolt left to go on holidays. He arranged for another orthopaedic surgeon to be available for contact if there were any problems. Prior to his departure, Dr Shadbolt did not return to the ward or ascertain the results of the wound swab. Dr Carey did not review the wound swab results and discharged Jake on 23 October 2015. Nursing staff were aware of the wound swab results from the time they arrived in both the email and the physical in-trays of the rehabilitation ward. The results were left in the in-tray for review by medical personnel.

Jake returned to the hospital for daily and then second daily dressings until 30 October 2015. He was told by nursing staff that he had a "Staph infection" and that the Keflex would knock it on its head.

By 7 November 2015, Jake began feeling generally unwell and experienced shivers and shakes. He saw his general practitioner, who was worried about an infection of the hip joint and referred him to the emergency department at the nearest hospital. At the hospital, Jake was diagnosed with a periprosthetic infection and underwent a right hip washout and debridement on 10 November 2015. Despite intravenous antibiotics, the infection returned. As a result, Jake underwent revision surgery on 1 December 2015.

The revision surgery was unsuccessful. Jake subsequently underwent a second revision operation, but has been left with significant disability in the form of pain and stiffness.

Legal Issues

Jake commenced proceedings in negligence against Dr Shadbolt, Dr Carey and the private hospital for failing promptly to diagnose and treat a deep-seated bacterial infection of his right hip.

Based upon orthopaedic expert evidence and infectious diseases opinion, Jake alleged that the persistent oozing about one week after the operation was consistent with secondary haemorrhage caused by infection. Dr Shadbolt ought to have considered a periprosthetic joint infection, taken a wound swab and then carried out a debridement or washout much sooner than occurred together with the administration of intravenous antibiotics. If this had eventuated, then Jake would have avoided the loss of his initial prosthesis and the need for two revision operations.

Expert orthopaedic opinions were obtained and relied on by the three defendants. While there was some dispute about the need to consider a deep-seated bacterial infection in the days prior to the wound swab being taken, there was little disagreement as to the need to act on the results once they were obtained. It was unsafe to consider Jake had a superficial infection when there was no evidence of surrounding cellulitis, which meant the discharge and ooze must have emanated from a deeper space. Oral Keflex was never going to contain a deep infection.

Dr Shadbolt agreed that, if he had known of the wound swab results, he would have considered a periprosthetic infection and would have arranged for urgent debridement and washout together with intravenous antibiotic therapy. The private hospital argued that it was not responsible for informing Dr Shadbolt or Dr Carey about the wound swab results as they were placed in the in-tray for Dr Carey to review. The results had also been emailed to Dr Carey. The fact that Dr Carey did not inspect the results was not the hospital's responsibility. Dr Carey argued that Dr Shadbolt should have followed up the results by telephoning nursing staff, coming in and reviewing Jake himself or ringing the pathology laboratory. Although there was an argument about responsibility for ascertaining the wound swab results, the most difficult issue in the case was whether earlier diagnosis and treatment would have avoided revision surgery, it being accepted that once Jake underwent two revision operations, the outcome was unlikely to be as good as with primary surgery.

The case is ongoing.

Discussion

The central issue in this case was communication. While the outcome with earlier diagnosis and surgery could be debated, there was no debate about the need for the wound swab results to have been communicated to Dr Shadbolt (or his locum) so that a decision on further treatment could be made. The bickering between the defendants about whose responsibility it was to ascertain the wound swab results and communicate them to Dr Shadbolt bordered on the farcical.

As the surgeon primarily responsible for Jake's treatment and postoperative management, and the person who ordered the test, Dr Shadbolt should have taken steps himself to review the results. On the other hand, it is not uncommon for surgeons to rely on nursing staff to inform them of key results, especially in a private hospital setting. The complicating factor in Jake's case was the involvement of an additional doctor in Jake's management, Dr Carey. The wound swab results were not forwarded to Dr Shadbolt by the laboratory, but were sent to the private hospital ward in which Jake was being treated as well as to Dr Carey (at the same address).

Nursing staff saw the results and left them in Dr Carey's in-tray. Nursing staff play a vital role in the management of patients. They are important members of the team. It is necessary for nursing and medical staff to communicate with each other rather than assuming one or the other will take responsibility. In this case, responsibility for communicating the wound results was shared. It was not appropriate for nursing staff to assume that Dr Carey would see the results or act on them. It was not appropriate for Dr Carey to assume that nursing staff would alert him to the results.

In the end, knowledge of the wound swab results fell between the cracks. The results were not appreciated or acted upon by anyone, to Jake's detriment.

Clinical Principles

Investigations are ordered every day in medical practice. Test results are received by hospitals and doctors every day. Sometimes, the results are seen by nursing staff, sometimes by doctors. Whatever the situation, a medical practice or hospital needs to have an effective system of follow-up with the patient and an effective system of communication between members of a treating team.

Rather than no communications being made in Jake's case, a proper system of communication and follow-up should have resulted in all three defendants knowing at about the same time the results of the wound swab. Dr Shadbolt should have had a proper system of follow-up of an investigation he ordered. Nursing staff at the private hospital should have had a system that mandates the results of a wound swab being reported to the treating surgeon, or to the treating rehabilitation physician, or both. Dr Carey should have checked his in-tray to ensure he was aware of results pertaining to patients he was managing.

CAUDA EQUINA SYNDROME

This chapter comprises three cases of cauda equina syndrome where the diagnosis was initially overlooked. We have written this chapter because delays in diagnosis of an acute cauda equina syndrome is a recurring theme in medical litigation.

The cauda equina (Latin for horse's tail) is a bundle of nerves at the base of the spine. These lumbar, sacral and coccygeal nerves supply pelvic muscles and organs, muscles of the lower limbs and sensation to the perineum and lower limbs. Cauda equina syndrome occurs when there is pressure on the nerves of the cauda equina. This is most commonly due to disc protrusion, infection or tumour. The diagnosis should be suspected when there is low back pain and clinical evidence of pelvic organ dysfunction with or without lower limb symptoms. The classic symptom of saddle anaesthesia may not be present in every case or may be a late development. Acute cauda equina syndrome is a neurosurgical emergency.

BACK PAIN WITH BOWEL AND BLADDER SYMPTOMS

HISTORY

Jim Shaw was a 54-year-old man who presented to his general practitioner, Dr Clive Curnow, with pain in the back and numbness in his left leg subsequent to a lifting strain.

Dr Curnow examined Jim and organised a computed tomogram (CT) scan, the results of which were to be reviewed with Jim two days later. The CT scan showed L5/S1 nerve root impingement on the right side by a disc-bar complex. There was evidence of degenerative disc disease. There was no description of any canal stenosis or of a central disc protrusion. When Dr Curnow next saw Jim his symptoms had worsened. Jim now experienced numbness to the testicles, right buttock and right thigh to the knee. Although the correct diagnosis was acute cauda equina syndrome for which immediate neurosurgical review was indicated, Dr Curnow arranged a routine appointment with a neurosurgeon.

Overnight Jim had difficulty emptying his bowels and bladder, and presented to the emergency department at the nearby teaching hospital. No active treatment was provided.

When his symptoms had not abated six days later Jim returned to Dr Curnow. Even though Jim now had bowel and bladder dysfunction in addition to numbness in his testicles and lower limbs, Dr Curnow did not arrange immediate neurosurgical review.

Eight days later Jim was eventually seen by the neurosurgeon, who ordered an urgent MRI scan of the lumbosacral spine. This demonstrated a central disc protrusion likely compressing the cauda equina. Jim underwent urgent decompressive surgery. Unsurprisingly, Jim never recovered normal bowel or bladder function.

Legal Issues

Jim sought compensation for the consequences of delayed diagnosis of acute cauda equina syndrome. Dr Curnow admitted liability and the case was settled before trial.

Discussion

Dr Curnow did not understand that Jim's symptoms could not be explained by the isolated L5/S1 nerve root compression on the right side. He failed to appreciate that Jim had symptoms in both lower limbs and in the perineum which could not be due to L5/S1 nerve root compression on the right side.

Numbness of the testicles involved lower sacral nerves (i.e. below the level of L5/S1). Numbness of the buttocks and thigh involved nerves arising above L5/S1. Compression of the cauda equina was not appreciated on the CT scan. If Dr Curnow had considered carefully the neuroanatomy involved in Jim's symptoms he would have realised the extent of Jim's pathology. He ought to have considered a central disc bulge in view of the recent history of lifting, especially in someone with degenerative disease of his spinal column. If Jim had undergone surgery sooner than was the case, permanent bowel and bladder dysfunction would likely have been eliminated or reduced.

Both Dr Curnow and the hospital doctor were somehow reassured by the CT scan report. Neither seemed to have considered that the CT scan was merely an aid to diagnosis and that Jim's history indicated neuropathology beyond L5/S1. Further investigation by way of an MRI scan was required.

It has been often said that if one listens to the patient's story they will tell you the diagnosis. Each of the practitioners managing Jim had not considered examining his perineum despite his clinical symptoms. If they had examined Jim's perineum they would have detected reduced sensation, which would have directed their attention to the lower sacral nerves and the need for urgent neurosurgical review.

Clinical Principles

An understanding of neuroanatomy is essential to evaluation of neurological symptoms. Cauda equina syndrome must be considered when a patient presents with back pain, pelvic organ dysfunction and lower limb symptoms. Acute cauda equina syndrome is a neurosurgical emergency. A negative CT scan does not contradict symptoms which indicate cauda equina syndrome. A negative CT scan is no more reassuring than the absence of saddle anaesthesia. Delayed treatment of acute cauda equina syndrome increases the risk of permanent disability.

SACRAL PAIN WITH EVIDENCE OF INFECTION

HISTORY

Freya Cummings, aged 60 years, had suffered intermittent back pain for over a decade. The disability had always involved the mid lumbar area with pain radiating down the left leg, and this discomfort always occurred after lifting.

Freya attended her usual general practitioner, Dr John Penklis, with acute back pain radiating down the right thigh. The pain was located in the sacral area and was boring in nature. In addition to this, there was a change in her bowel habit. Dr Penklis considered that Freya had suffered a pinched nerve of similar aetiology to her longstanding problem. He prescribed analgesics.

The disability settled to a manageable degree until Freya contacted Dr Penklis six months later with a flare-up of similar symptoms. The practice secretary told Freya that Dr Penklis was unavailable and that she should recommence the previously prescribed medication. Three days later Freya phoned the practice again, and once more received the same reply.

As a result of her persistent pain and the inability to obtain an appointment with her general practitioner, Freya attended the local hospital that day where she was seen by an intern who recorded a temperature of 37.5°C, and noted bilateral sensory deficits at L1 and S1, an ESR of 56 mm/h (reference <30 mm/h) and a CRP of 258 mg/L (reference <5 mg/L).

The intern concluded that Freya was suffering from a urinary tract infection and prescribed trimethoprim 300 mg daily for three days.

Freya presented to the hospital three days later with the same symptoms and with the addition of numbness and loss of power of the right leg and frequent watery bowel movements. She was unable to pass urine. A resident medical officer who assessed her made the meaningless diagnosis of low back pain, prescribed analgesics and discharged her home.

On the insistence of her husband, Freya did not return home, and later that day an orthopaedic registrar suggested that she had either a prolapsed disc or an epidural abscess and that she needed an urgent MRI scan. This investigation was not available at the local hospital, and the MRI was scheduled at a tertiary referral centre 20 kilometres away for the following day. Freya spent the night on a trolley at the local hospital. The MRI scan the next day revealed an epidural abscess, for which she underwent urgent decompressive surgery.

Freya now suffers with incomplete paraplegia, recurrent urinary tract infections, faecal and urinary incontinence, anxiety and depression.

LEGAL ISSUES

Freya brought proceedings against Dr Penklis and the local hospital for the consequences of delayed diagnosis of a spinal epidural abscess compressing the cauda equina.

Both the plaintiff and the two defendants obtained expert reports from general practitioners, emergency physicians, infectious diseases physicians and neurosurgeons. The dispute between the general practitioners centred on the change in Freya's usual presenting symptoms with back pain. The pain was not associated with lifting and involved the contralateral limb. It was also associated with unusual symptoms. Dr Penklis obtained general practitioner support for his assumption that the pain was likely to be associated with degenerative spinal disease so that it was reasonable to treat it conservatively. As the pain abated, his treatment approach was justified. The expert was less robust in his views about Dr Penklis' conduct six months later.

There was no real contest about the local hospital's treatment. Experts accepted that the diagnosis of a urinary tract infection was unsustainable. The contest was whether the delay made any significance to Freya's outcome.

The case is ongoing.

Discussion

Dr Penklis had cared for Freya for many years. When he was unavailable to see Freya, on two occasions the practice secretary advised Freya to continue analgesic therapy. She did not offer an appointment for urgent review with another practitioner and did not advise Freya to go the local hospital. First, it was inappropriate for the secretary to provide clinical advice. Her behaviour reflected poorly on the training and education of staff by the general practitioners responsible for patient care.

Secondly it was inappropriate to not suggest review with another doctor in the practice or at the hospital when Freya had ongoing pain and other symptoms. There must have been a responsibility, in the obligation to provide continuity of care, to arrange for the patient to see a colleague if the usual practitioner was unavailable over several days.

The hospital intern observed neurological deficits and evidence of infection, yet did not seek the advice of a senior colleague. A resident medical officer at the same hospital ignored Freya's inability to pass urine and tried to send her home. The orthopaedic registrar recognised the need for an urgent MRI scan, yet this was deferred until the following day. There are often logistical issues in regional centres in relation to investigations. Twenty kilometres was hardly a barrier to timely investigation in light of Freya's persistent and progressive problems. By the time Freya saw the neurosurgeon, the prospect of any reduction in the severity of her neurological deficits was remote.

Freya was denied the chance of a better outcome because of avoidable delays in diagnosis.

Clinical Principles

Doctors must be sufficiently astute to identify changes in the pattern of presentation of patients with long-term conditions. Such changes may be very important. As here, they may represent the onset of a new, serious problem. The failure to recognise the significance of a new set of problems may have resulted in the delay in diagnosing the spinal epidural abscess and acute cauda equina syndrome.

The consequences of a delay in diagnosis of acute cauda equina syndrome cannot be understated. The diagnosis should have been considered when Freya had persistent sacral pain, urinary retention, lower limb numbness and weakness and evidence of infection. But it does not need a full hand of symptoms to be considered as a possible diagnosis. Good medical practice is about prevention and not treating conditions when they are blindingly obvious and beyond hope for recovery.

BACK PAIN AND URINARY RETENTION

History

Jean Tregear was aged 38 at the time she presented to her local hospital with low back pain, mainly left-sided sciatica and difficulty voiding. She had a previous low back disorder resulting from a work injury seven years prior to the presentation. She was seen by Dr Moses Mweratua in the emergency department. Her back was examined; she was given crutches and analgesia, and asked to return if the problem became worse. No neurological examination was performed by Dr Mweratua. The diagnosis was of mechanical back pain. A letter was written to her general practitioner, Dr Irwin Halloran, whom she saw after two days.

Dr Halloran performed a cursory examination and arranged an MRI scan that was performed two days later. He did not perform a neurological examination. The report stated, "At L4/5 there appears to be a mild left sided disc protrusion probably with some restrictions at the lateral left recess and impressions on the left side descending L5 nerve root. At L5/S1 there is a large sequestered disc protrusion mainly on the left side with compression of the left sided roots particularly in the descending left sided S1 nerve root." The report was poorly worded. It suggested obliquely with the words "mainly on the left side" that the disc protrusion affected both sides. This was compatible with the fact that Jean had other than left leg symptoms. Dr Halloran referred Jean to a local neurosurgeon, who fortuitously was able to see her in a week. No sense of urgency was conveyed by Dr Halloran to either Jean or the neurosurgeon.

One week later Jean saw a neurosurgeon who immediately diagnosed her with acute cauda equina syndrome and performed urgent decompressive surgery that day. The neurosurgical record referred to, "Excruciating left leg pain, saddle hypoaesthesia, incomplete emptying of her bladder, significant urinary urgency, absent left Achilles reflex." None of this history had found its way into Dr Halloran's or the local hospital's record even though it was available to be elicited.

Despite the surgical intervention, Jean did not recover normal neurological function.

Legal Issues

Jean sued Dr Halloran and the local hospital responsible for Dr Mweratua for the permanent impairment secondary to the delayed diagnosis and treatment of cauda equina syndrome. The radiologist who wrote the ambiguous and somewhat misleading report on the MRI scan was not joined.

Expert opinions were obtained from general practitioners, emergency specialists and neurosurgeons. The local hospital attempted to argue that, if Dr Mweratua had performed a neurological examination, no abnormalities would have been found. It argued that the symptoms recorded by the neurosurgeon were not present at the time of Dr Mweratua's examination because if they had been, he would have recorded them. It was reasonable to treat the problem as an acute exacerbation of a pre-existing long-term problem and to refer Jean back to her general practitioner for further management.

The general practitioner retained by Dr Halloran argued that he ordered the correct investigation and that there was no need for greater urgency given Jean's history of back pain. Referral to a neurosurgeon was consistent with proper professional practice. It was not explained how it was reasonable to ignore the urinary symptoms or to fail to conduct a neurological examination.

The case is ongoing.

Discussion

Prior to the neurosurgical consultation no one had examined Jean carefully to detect neurological signs. In light of the absence of the same history elicited by the neurosurgeon, it is doubtful that Jean was interrogated properly about any neurological symptoms. Further, given what the neurosurgeon found just before surgery, it was likely some deficits would have been detected if Jean had been examined thoroughly and if her history and signs were considered thoughtfully.

There are various ways to detect incomplete bladder emptying such as by ultrasound. If one is working in a remote setting without an ultrasound one can ask the patient to void and then use a catheter to measure the volume of residual urine. There is no need to wait for an ultrasound or MRI scan to diagnose incomplete bladder emptying. It does not appear that the history of voiding difficulty was explored in great detail or thought to be connected to the low back pain. It is always much more likely that there is a single explanation for presenting symptoms rather than multiple independent diagnoses. Neither Dr Mweratua or Dr Halloran reasoned in this way.

Jean's MRI scan report was confusing as it described features "mainly" on the left side. If the report had been more specific and had included the word "central" this may have prompted Dr Halloran to refer Jean urgently for neurosurgical review. Thoughtful reporting and careful use of words is vital to effective communication between practitioners. In this particular case, central disc protrusion was more likely to affect the innervation to the bladder than was unilateral protrusion. Even with the ambiguous wording of the report, common sense should have dictated consideration of a central protrusion.

The problem with this case, and the other two, is that the symptoms were complex and not related to a single region supplied by a sciatic nerve. The three patients did not have classic saddle anaesthesia (or at least recorded by anyone other than the neurosurgeon). This may have allayed the doctors' anxiety about a possible acute cauda equina syndrome. Their history-taking and examinations seem to suggest they had little anxiety about the presence of the condition.

A detailed understanding of neuroanatomy remains important. Modern teaching encourages students to have a sense of inquiry. Such a sense of inquiry with working knowledge of neuroanatomy should have allowed Jean and the other two patients to have been correctly assessed sooner.

Clinical Principles

When a condition known to be a neurosurgical emergency is considered as a working or even differential diagnosis, investigation and treatment must be undertaken urgently. There seemed to have been no sense of urgency in Jean's case (or the other two). It was a matter of coincidence that she was seen by a neurosurgeon within a week of the MRI scan. The more quickly that a possible cauda equina syndrome is diagnosed, the better the prognosis and the less the risk of permanent neurological damage. Emergencies are just that: things need to be done urgently. Even though acute cauda equina syndrome is known to be a neurosurgical emergency, it seems that many doctors have disparate views on what an emergency means and how fast one needs to move. In addition, it seems that some doctors, even in emergency departments, continue to be unfamiliar with the clinical features of this condition or cognisant of what investigations are required to aid in this diagnosis.

BLADDER CANCER

HISTORY

At the age of 54, primary school teacher Ahmad Abbas noticed blood in his urine. He hoped it was nothing to worry about and that it would go away. After four days, his urine was still discoloured and he developed dysuria. He decided to see his general practitioner, Dr Sadiq Mahmood.

On 22 September 2011, Dr Mahmood ordered a number of investigations, including urine cytology. This demonstrated abnormal urothelial cells suggestive of a high-grade transitional cell carcinoma (TCC). An ultrasound demonstrated a posterior bladder mass 70 mm × 61 mm × 19 mm with hypervascularity and a configuration typical of TCC. As a result of the investigations, Dr Mahmood referred Ahmad to urologist Dr Andy McIntyre.

Ahmad lived with his wife and family in a regional centre near Melbourne. Dr McIntyre was one of four urologists practising in the private and public health systems in the area.

Ahmad consulted Dr McIntyre on 7 October 2011. He told Ahmad that he had a TCC of his bladder and advised him to undergo cystoscopy, biopsy and a bilateral retrograde pyelogram.

On 17 October 2011, Ahmad underwent cystoscopy, resection biopsy and a bilateral retrograde pyelogram at a local private hospital. At operation, Dr McIntyre found that almost half of the bladder was occupied by multifocal papillary TCC. Subsequent histopathological examination of the biopsy specimen demonstrated a high-grade papillary grade 3 TCC invading through the muscularis propria of the bladder with a maximum invasion thickness of 5 mm, but without any vascular invasion.

At a follow-up consultation, Dr McIntyre ordered a CT scan of Ahmad's chest and abdomen for staging purposes. There was no evidence of lymph node or distant metastases.

On 25 October 2011, Ahmad again consulted Dr McIntyre for the purpose of advice about further management of the TCC. During the consultation, Dr McIntyre advised Ahmad that he was an appropriate candidate for radical surgical treatment of the TCC because of the absence of any metastases. He advised Ahmad that the treatment options were chemotherapy, radiation therapy or a radical cystectomy. Dr McIntyre recommended a radical cystectomy as he believed the cancer could be eradicated given the absence of secondaries. He went on to advise Ahmad that, if he chose radical cystectomy, then he had two options in relation to the diversion of his urine – simple incontinence ileostomy or a neobladder constructed from his ileum. Dr McIntyre informed Ahmad that the risks associated with the neobladder operation were incontinence, mucous plugging and urinary retention. He informed Ahmad that there was a slightly higher complication rate with the neobladder because it was a more complex operation than ileal diversion. Dr McIntyre recommended neobladder formation.

After careful consideration of Dr McIntyre's advice and discussing the options with his wife, Ahmad opted for a radical cystectomy with pelvic lymph node dissection and continent urinary diversion through the formation of a neobladder. Ahmad went ahead with the operation at the local private hospital on 30 October 2011.

During the operation, Ahmad's ileum became ischaemic and required resection on two occasions. Dr McIntyre abandoned neobladder formation and opted for an ileostomy for urinary diversion. After the operation, Ahmad required further surgery to resect infarcted small bowel and mesentery. He remained seriously ill. Dr McIntyre asked for a second opinion from his urology colleague, Professor Hamish MacDonald.

On 3 February 2012, Ahmad was operated on by Professor MacDonald, who performed a left percutaneous nephrostomy and a right open circle nephrostomy. As he was suspected of suffering abdominal sepsis, Professor MacDonald ordered a CT scan of the abdomen. This was performed on 30 April 2012, and revealed possible liver secondaries. A liver biopsy confirmed the presence of hepatic metastases.

On 20 August 2012, Ahmad died prematurely from metastatic TCC of the bladder. He left behind his wife and two sons.

Legal Issues

In 2014 Ahmad's wife, Raina, sued Dr McIntyre in negligence on her own behalf and on behalf of Ahmad's estate. She also claimed damages under Lord Campbell's Act for her and her children's loss and the expectation of receiving pecuniary benefits had Ahmad survived.

The case was supported by the opinions of two urologists and an oncologist. It was accepted that, at the time of the initial cystoscopy and biopsy on 17 October 2011, Ahmad had microscopic liver secondaries and thus was always going to have a negative prognosis. There was no criticism of the radiologist, who did not identify any metastases at the time he reported his findings of the staging CT scan. Dr McIntyre could not have known that his recommendation for surgery with curative intent was never likely to succeed. Instead, the case focused on a different issue.

At the time Dr McIntyre recommended a radical cystectomy with neobladder construction, he was not permitted to perform such major surgery in the public hospital system because of an unacceptable morbidity and mortality rate. A clinical audit had been conducted in the public hospital system which effectively found that Dr McIntyre did not possess the skills or experience to perform major surgery such as a radical cystectomy and neobladder construction. Notwithstanding this limitation on his practice, and his knowledge that the public hospital system offered greater facilities, services and backup than the local private hospital for the performance of complex surgery, Dr McIntyre went ahead and recommended that Ahmad's surgery be conducted at the local private hospital. The plaintiff's experts were critical of this decision.

Dr McIntyre did not disclose to Ahmad and his wife that he had any restrictions on the type of surgery he was able to perform in the public system. They were not told about the surgical backup available in the private hospital in the event of complications or that there was an increased incidence of serious complications in Dr McIntyre's hands. Ahmad's wife alleged that Ahmad would not have consented to the operation, and that she would have ensured that he did not consent to the operation, if such information had been provided by Dr McIntyre. She argued that Ahmad would have obtained a second opinion from another urologist, which ultimately would have led to the surgery being performed in the public sector by an approved urologist.

The expert urological opinion accepted that these complications were less likely to have occurred in the hands of a more experienced and skilled urologist performing the surgery in the public system. As a result of the complications, Ahmad suffered major intraabdominal and general sepsis. He was unable to undergo chemotherapy when the liver secondaries were identified. If he had undergone surgery without complications, the lesions would have been correctly identified as secondaries. He would have undergone chemotherapy earlier and his survival would have improved by a number of years. There was, however, no dispute that his prognosis was poor even with uncomplicated major surgery.

The real contest was between the competing oncological opinions about Ahmad's survival if he had been able to undergo earlier chemotherapy for metastatic disease. The opinions ranged from additional survival of months to up to three years with a reasonable quality of life.

As it turned out, Ahmad and his family endured months of pain and suffering beyond that which would be expected for a diagnosis of TCC of the bladder with hepatic secondaries. Ahmad's wife alleged that this ordeal was solely the responsibility of Dr McIntyre for recommending and performing an operation he had no business performing.

The quantum of the case was significantly circumscribed because of Ahmad's prognosis even with proper treatment.

The matter settled at mediation.

DISCUSSION

The case highlights the need for medical practitioners to act within their level of competency.

It also reinforces the need for a doctor to accept the umpire's call when there has been an objective evaluation by peers of his or her competence. It is impossible to fathom how Dr McIntyre thought he had the skills and experience to perform major, complex surgery at a regional private hospital when he was not permitted to perform such surgery in the public hospital system where there was a range of surgical specialties available to assist, including other urologists, colorectal surgeons and an intensive care unit.

In addition, the case stresses the need for patients to be informed of any restrictions on their treating doctors' right to practise. The question whether a patient should be entitled to this type of information is very difficult to answer. If his lack of competence had been referred to the Australian Health Practitioner Regulation Agency (AHPRA) or the Health Professional Councils Authority (HPCA), it is likely that they would have been critical of Dr McIntyre's decision to perform such an operation when his peers had concluded that he did not have sufficient competence to do so.

While there were no formal restrictions on Dr McIntyre's right to practise from a medical registration perspective, the fact that he had undergone a clinical audit following an elevated rate of complications for the very surgery he was advising Ahmad to undergo ought to have triggered a realisation on his part that Ahmad would undoubtedly attach significance to the information in deciding to consent to the proposed operation. Dr McIntyre probably thought he had no legal obligation to pass on the information. He might have been worried it could be detrimental to his ability to derive an income if he had to tell all his patients of his complication rates.

The case also raises questions about credentialling of doctors at private hospitals. In order to operate at a private hospital, a surgeon needs to apply and provide information about the types of operation he or she proposes to perform at the hospital. There should have been clearer communication about the type of surgery that Dr McIntyre was able to perform. More stringent bylaws for private hospitals may have ensured that information about Dr McIntyre's problems with performing major urological surgery was forthcoming.

Between 2011 and 2016, there were 43,256 notifications of concern regarding the health, performance and conduct of health practitioners lodged with AHPRA and HPCA. 11.9% of the notifications were made by fellow practitioners. Fellow practitioners were a common source of notifications about advertising and titles, but fewer than 10% of all performance notifications were lodged by fellow practitioners. (1)

The adoption of mandatory reporting requirements may improve patient outcomes. Other specialists may have been aware of Dr McIntyre's practice of undertaking adventurous surgery in the private health system, but may have been unaware of their capacity to do anything about it.

Furthermore, it is strange that AHPRA was unaware of the results of the investigation into Dr McIntyre's morbidity and mortality rates. This was likely to have been relevant information to disclose when applying for registration renewal. The reason for nondisclosure may well have been the wording used in the renewal process as to what matters should be disclosed. This may require careful review.

In addition, there may often be a demarcation line between the public and private health systems. There may be attitudes that anything that occurs outside the public hospital system is a matter for the particular doctor and the private hospital administration. It is unclear whether the public hospital contacted AHPRA or the HPCA to complain about Dr McIntyre's complication rates. While whistleblowing may be an unpleasant step to take, patient safety is the central determinant of what to do. After the clinical audit, there should have been an information exchange with private hospitals and with regulatory authorities.

What eventuated was a mismatch between Dr McIntyre's skill level and the facilities and services available at the local private hospital at which he was performing major surgery. If medical practitioners do not report concerns to AHPRA, then it becomes difficult to have proper supervision and review of clinical performance. Not all patients make complaints. Not all patients know how to make complaints. The practice of medicine would be enhanced by heed being given to mandatory reporting requirements and the need to communicate between the public and private systems. The responsibility of AHPRA to assess a doctor's performance does not relieve hospitals from properly reviewing a doctor's performance on a regular basis. (2)

Clinical Principles

From time to time, a medical practitioner's competency may be called into question. This is not simply a matter of a difference of opinion, but repeated errors in judgment, a cluster of cases with bad outcomes or more obvious irrational behaviour and impairment. It is a sensitive, troubling and stressful aspect of medical practice. Questions are thrown up about whether to turn a blind eye or take steps to report concerns to administration or regulatory authorities. Systems and regulations should be in place to manage this most difficult area. Early recognition, discussion and reporting may result in less harm to patients and fewer cases going to court.

References

(1) Bismark, M., et al., 2018. Eyes and ears on patient safety. Sources of notifications about the health, performance and conduct of health practitioners. J. Patient Saf.

(2) See for example the recommendations of Furness "Review of Documentary Material in Relation to the Appointment of Dr Gayed, Management of Complaints about Dr Gayed and Compliance with Conditions Imposed on Dr Gayed by Local Health Districts", 21 January 2019.

PENILE CANCER

History

Boris Umanoff suffered from psoriasis. This was managed with antiinflammatory drugs and ointments together with intermittent immunosuppressive therapy. Boris, who was fair-skinned, regularly underwent a "skin check" with a dermatologist to look for skin cancers. He had undergone ultraviolet B (UVB) treatment. The psoriasis had from time to time affected his penis. His penile psoriasis routinely responded to Daivobet 50/500 ointment, which contained a vitamin D derivative, calcipotriol, and a corticosteroid, betamethasone. Boris had an active sex life with his wife.

In May 2011, Boris noticed a raised scab on the dorsum of the shaft of his penis. He thought the lesion was a recurrence of psoriasis and treated it with Daivobet ointment. The lesion did not go away. He used other creams and ointments, including pawpaw cream, to no avail. His penis was mildly tender and occasionally bled slightly on contact. In August 2011, Boris's general practitioner, Dr Selwyn Clark, referred him to Dr Gregory Tan, a dermatologist, for advice and treatment. At the time of the referral, Boris was taking methotrexate 25 mg weekly and prednisone 5 mg daily for the psoriasis.

Boris consulted Dr Tan on 30 August 2011. He performed a skin check and identified a worrying lesion on Boris's right leg, which he biopsied. The biopsy subsequently demonstrated a squamous cell carcinoma (SCC).

He then attended to the penile lesion. Dr Tan's notes recorded no history of the lesion other than "wart on penis". There was no history about its duration, whether it was associated with any symptoms, such as bleeding or itchiness, whether it was painful, etc. There was no history in relation to whether Boris had multiple sexual partners or a new sexual partner, which was relevant to the development of a new human papilloma viral (HPV) infection. He did not record that Boris had been treated with methotrexate and prednisone for psoriasis, or that Boris had undergone UVB treatment. His notes simply recorded that he diagnosed the lesion as a wart virus for which he recommended a wart ointment. He reported back to Dr Clark in those terms. He also referred Boris to a plastic surgeon for wide excision of the lesion on the leg.

Boris subsequently saw Dr Clark for a number of issues, including the so-called wart on the penis. Dr Clark prescribed wart treatment in the form of podophyllotoxin cream in accordance with the recommendations of Dr Tan.

After the SCC of the right leg was treated, Boris returned to Dr Tan on 11 December 2011 for a check-up in relation to the right leg wound. He also pointed out the penile lesion, which he said had grown in size, was bleeding more often and was inflamed. Dr Tan examined Boris's penis and noticed that it was inflamed and had spread to the base of the penis. He diagnosed an infection secondary to the use of the podophyllotoxin treatment and prescribed an antibiotic. Boris returned on multiple occasions to see Dr Clark, who continued to treat the penile lesion as a wart with secondary inflammation and infection from the podophyllotoxin treatment. Ultimately, at Boris's urging, Dr Clark referred him back to Dr Tan.

On 30 April 2012, Dr Tan biopsied the penile lesion. By that time it involved the whole of the dorsal surface of the shaft of the penis. The biopsy was reported as showing a well-differentiated SCC with overlying Bowen's disease. Dr Tan referred Boris to a urologist specialising in penile cancer, Professor Adam Turner, who recommended a total penectomy because of the extent of the SCC. He advised Boris that he may have been able to save his penis if the SCC had been diagnosed earlier.

On 27 July 2012, Boris underwent a total penectomy with perineal urethrostomy for treatment of the penile SCC. He also underwent bilateral inguinal lymph node dissection, which resulted in bilateral lower limb lymphoedema. Histopathological examination of the penis revealed SCC, Bowen's disease and some changes consistent with prior HPV infection.

Boris was devastated by the outcome. When Dr Tan initially advised him that he had HPV infection, there was considerable finger-pointing and disharmony with his wife over who was responsible for the HPV infection. Once that had settled, he was then confronted with treatment in the form of a total penectomy and a loss of all sexual relations with his wife. On top of that, he had painful disabling lymphoedema. His capacity to undertake tasks at home and at work was seriously compromised. Given the histopathological findings of past HPV infection, the question of its origin remained uncertain.

Legal Issues

Boris commenced legal proceedings in negligence against Dr Tan. Based upon the expert opinion of an independent dermatologist, Boris argued that Dr Tan should have biopsied the penile lesion at the first consultation or no later than the second consultation when he returned with an inflamed, spreading lesion on the shaft of his penis. It was argued that Dr Tan should have attached significance to the fact that Boris was on immunosuppressive therapy for his psoriasis as such therapy may promote carcinogenesis. In addition, he ought to have been aware that UVB therapy increased the risk of skin cancers.

Dr Tan made no enquiry in relation to Boris's sexual history. He did not describe the lesion or attach significance to what Boris said was a raised, non-itchy, tender lesion that occasionally bled on contact. The expert dermatologist was of the opinion that a reasonable dermatologist could not have been confident that the lesion was a wart or even psoriasis without taking a biopsy. It was not a diagnosis that could be safely made by simple examination. Even if it were reasonable to make a provisional diagnosis of a wart with associated psoriasis, that diagnosis was patently untenable a matter of months later when the lesion had not responded to wart treatment and, in fact, had become worse.

The expert was of the view that Dr Tan at least ought to have considered Bowen's disease, which is a carcinoma in situ occurring within the epithelium on the penile shaft. Bowen's disease presents as a solitary, dull-red plaque with areas of crusting and oozing. It may be associated with HPV and, if untreated, may result in SCC. The dermatologist considered that, given the confounding effect of psoriasis, it could not have been safe for Dr Tan to assume that the lesion was due to psoriasis or HPV. A biopsy was appropriate.

Boris also obtained an opinion from a urologist, who, as with the dermatologist, considered that, if the lesion had been biopsied at the first or second presentation, the penile cancer would have been smaller in size and amenable to organ preservation surgery. Boris also would have undergone dynamic sentinel inguinal node biopsy rather than radical lymph node dissection so that the likelihood of lymphoedema would have been substantially lower.

Dr Tan served his own independent dermatology opinion. Somewhat unusually, Dr Tan asserted that he recalled the consultations with Boris. He asserted by way of assumptions to his experts that he performed a proper examination of the penis, took an admirable history and excluded an SCC. He maintained that, as an expert dermatologist, he was well aware of the appearance of an SCC and would have diagnosed it had it genuinely been present. He also asserted that, after the initial consultation, he had referred Boris back to Dr Clark to manage the treatment of the wart so that he did not assume any ongoing responsibility for the treatment of the lesion. This assertion was contrary to Dr Tan's prescription of an antibiotic at the second consultation. The dermatology opinion also argued that Boris's outcome would have been the same with earlier diagnosis, although the basis for that assertion was unclear.

The matter settled at mediation.

Discussion

This case again demonstrates the importance of taking and recording a proper history. If Dr Tan had taken a history about the duration of the lesion, whether it had responded to anti-psoriasis treatment, Boris's sexual history, his immunosuppressive therapy and treatment with UVB and his age, he should have considered Bowen's disease and associated SCC as differential diagnoses. While Dr Tan argued that he had taken an adequate history and that his examination ruled out the presence of SCC, his records did not remotely support the argument.

Dr Tan's defence was also that he would have diagnosed the SCC if it had been present. He knew what they looked like. This represented a failure to recognise the limits of his ability. Doctors are not infallible. Unrealistic confidence has no place in the management of patients. At the very least, Dr Tan should have revised his opinion at the second consultation and biopsied the penile lesion. While he may have been distracted by the SCC on Boris's right leg, this did not pardon any lack of attention or superficiality in his assessment of the penile lesion.

Finally, the case highlights the need for frankness in evaluating one's professional conduct. Mistakes are made in clinical practice. There is nothing wrong with admitting that a mistake has been made. By the time matters go to lawyers and litigation is commenced, the reality of clinical practice is lost and parties often engage in sophistry to deny liability. Assumptions are often put to experts based on a doctor's belief that it is virtually impossible to have made such a simple mistake as omitting to take a history of a key point or failing to order a relevant test. Boris was dismayed by Dr Tan's assertions about what took place during the relevant consultations. Litigation simply aggravates an injury, and leads to professional anguish. Apologies and the communication of honest mistakes go a long way to avoiding litigation or in reducing the stress of litigation.

Clinical Principles

Proper history taking and record keeping are the cornerstones of competent medical practice. Dr Tan's diagnosis was at odds with the story Boris endeavoured to explain to him. Diagnoses are not always made by clinical examination alone. Time pressures may tempt a practitioner to proceed straight to an examination. Examination follows a history. The next step in clinical evaluation is to consider all the features of the history and examination in order to formulate a provisional diagnosis and differential diagnoses. These diagnoses are then tested by relevant investigations and treatments.

The provisional diagnosis must be questioned if the course of an illness is inconsistent with an initial diagnosis.

LEG WEAKNESS

HISTORY

Stan Crockett was born in 1938. In July 2012, at the age of 74, his general practitioner Dr Toby Cox referred him to neurologist Dr Gulab Ahmed to investigate a five-week history of increasing weakness and numbness in the right lower limb with similar mild symptoms in the left lower limb. Dr Cox ordered a CT scan of Stan's spine, which showed degenerative disease, but nothing to suggest spinal cord pathology or impingement on any nerve roots.

Dr Cox's referring letter included the results of the CT scan. Dr Ahmed saw Stan three days later. He found significant sensory and motor abnormalities, particularly in the right leg. Nerve conduction studies demonstrated bilateral lower limb sensory and motor dysfunction. In a letter to Dr Cox after the consultation, Dr Ahmed said that Stan's problems included mild, right foot drop; antalgic gait; profound sensory impairment to pinprick and vibration (presumably bilateral); and absent knee and ankle jerks with depressed deep tendon reflexes in the right upper limb.

He diagnosed severe polyneuropathy, possibly axonal in nature. Dr Ahmed advised Dr Cox that Stan needed to be investigated to look for the cause of the neuropathy, including a lumbar puncture. Dr Ahmed did not order any radiological investigations; in particular he did not order a spinal MRI scan to ascertain whether there was a spinal cause for Stan's peripheral neurological symptoms. Dr Ahmed treated Stan on the assumption that it was a polyneuropathy requiring immunoglobulin therapy and corticosteroid therapy.

Stan deteriorated "despite" the immunoglobulin and steroid therapy to the point of requiring a rollator frame, but still managed to mobilise independently when he next saw Dr Ahmed in October 2012. Stan had bilateral severe foot drop and was unable to stand unassisted without his rollator frame. His sensory impairment was unchanged in three months. Dr Ahmed still did not have a cause for the polyneuropathy, which he explained in a letter to Dr Cox as being very resistant to all forms of therapy, and one which did not explain the severe paraplegia that Stan developed over the previous one to two months.

A second opinion was obtained from another neurologist, who saw Stan in November 2012. At this consultation Stan had gross weakness in both legs, including hip flexion, knee extension and flexion, ankle dorsiflexion and plantar flexion. He had reduced tone in his legs, and absent reflexes and bilateral sensory changes. Motor evoked potentials indicated combined upper and lower motor neurone pathology, suggesting pyramidal pathology or conduction block at a proximal level. This second neurologist recommended that an MRI scan of the spinal cord be repeated. In fact no MRI scan had ever been performed. It was assumed that an MRI scan of the spine would have been performed as a matter of course to investigate Stan's presenting condition in July 2012.

An MRI scan of Stan's spine was eventually ordered, and was performed in December 2012. It demonstrated a 1.5 cm diameter uniformly enhancing lesion at T10/11 with oedema above and below the lesion. There was some early syrinx formation distal to the lesion. The radiologist thought it was a metastasis or a primary spinal tumour such as an ependymoma.

Stan was referred urgently to a neurosurgeon. He performed a laminectomy and resected the spinal cord tumour at T10–12. The spinal cord tumour was a histologically benign intramedullary schwannoma. When Stan was eventually discharged from hospital, he underwent extensive spinal rehabilitation. He remains a T8 paraplegic with significant disabilities.

Legal Issues

Stan commenced proceedings against Dr Ahmed in 2014. He alleged that Dr Ahmed was negligent in not ordering an MRI scan of his spine as part of the initial investigation of his bilateral lower limb symptoms and signs, resulting in avoidable neurologic deficits.

Stan served expert reports from two neurologists and one neurosurgeon. The neurologists were strongly of the opinion that central or spinal cord pathology should have been on the list of differential diagnoses at the initial consultation. Investigations were required to confirm or exclude such pathologies. As an MRI scan is more sensitive in picking up spinal cord lesions, it should have been the investigation of choice. If an MRI scan had been performed, then the schwannoma would have been diagnosed. The expert neurosurgeon considered that the tumour would have been capable of being resected. If this had transpired, Stan's neurological deficits would not have progressed from being able to ambulate without assistance to being restricted to a wheelchair.

Dr Ahmed called no expert evidence from a neurosurgeon to dispute these contentions. He did not serve any report from a neurologist justifying his failure to order an MRI scan of the spine.

The case highlights the problem of causation in medical negligence cases. Very often there is a clear breach of duty by a doctor, as here, but the breach of duty does not cause any difference to outcome. In Stan's case, there was clear evidence of progression of his condition from the time he first consulted Dr Ahmed to the time of his decompressive surgery. It was possible to identify what symptoms and signs would have been avoided with earlier surgery. That is not always the case.

The neurological and neurosurgical opinion was that the delay in diagnosis significantly contributed to the nature and extent of Stan's paraplegia. Up until the catastrophic deterioration in Stan's spinal cord function towards the end of Dr Ahmed's therapeutic relationship with Stan, there had been a gradual deterioration in his neurological deficits.

Stan would not have avoided all of his permanent neurological symptoms and signs if the tumour had been resected earlier. This is because earlier surgery would more likely than not have stopped progression of his problems, but would not have eradicated them.

Causation and quantification of damages required a comparison between Stan's neurological problems at presentation to Dr Ahmed in July 2012 compared with those he had after his surgery. The contemporaneous records indicated that he progressed to obvious paraplegia in the five-month period.

If the case had gone to trial, Stan was likely to prove that he would have avoided his marked T8 paraplegia. At worst, he would have been left with a mild right foot drop, difficulty walking and a profound bilateral sensory impairment. These impairments were clearly much less severe initially than at the time of the surgery.

The matter settled at mediation.

Discussion

Dr Ahmed did not seriously dispute that he should have ordered a spinal MRI scan at the time of Stan's initial presentation. He was under the mistaken impression that the CT scan of the lumbar spine, performed in July at Dr Cox's request, was an MRI scan of the spine.

This mistake highlights a recurring theme in medical malpractice claims – an assumption that another practitioner has taken, or will take, an important investigative or therapeutic step. Some doctors assume a history taken by a predecessor is accurate and neglect to elicit their own. Some assume that obvious causes have already been investigated, as here. General practitioners may think that the specialist to whom they have referred a patient will assume responsibility for investigating a condition, and therefore are relieved of the burden to think about investigating a problem further.

Dr Ahmed assumed that an MRI scan had already been performed. This caused him to believe that Stan had an unusual polyneuropathy. It caused a five-month delay in diagnosis and treatment. Making assumptions without checking if they are well-founded can be dangerous. While the vast majority of these oversights will not cause any harm to a patient, occasionally, as in Stan's case, they do. Assumptions should always be verified.

In his initial letter to Dr Cox, Dr Ahmed indicated that spinal pathology needed to be excluded with a lumbar puncture. He would not have ordered a lumbar puncture on its own to investigate spinal pathology unless he already believed a spinal MRI scan had been performed.

According to the expert neurologists relied on by Stan, it was unreasonable for Dr Ahmed to have made a provisional diagnosis of a severe sensorimotor polyneuropathy without first investigating and excluding a central cause for Stan's presentation.

One dictum in medical practice is that common things occur commonly. It could not possibly represent proper practice for a neurologist to jump to the conclusion that there was a peripheral (less likely) cause without excluding a central or proximal (more likely) cause for Stan's illness. This is not to say that a schwannoma is a common occurrence, but rather that proximal pathology was at least equally likely or more likely than an obscure peripheral polyneuropathy to explain Stan's presenting symptoms and signs.

Clinical Principles

It is always appropriate to include potentially serious diagnoses in the list of differential diagnoses to explain a set of clinical features. This is especially important when there might be curative treatment for a particular diagnosis (in this case excision of a histologically benign spinal tumour).

It is always correct to question an initial diagnosis (of one's own, or that of another practitioner), especially if the course of a disease is not typical for the initial diagnosis.

It is never correct to assume that another individual has performed all the appropriate investigations, without checking that those investigations have in fact been performed.

Care must be taken when interpreting results to make sure that the conclusion relates to the test performed (in this case CT scan), and not to the test that should have been performed (MRI was indicated).

LACERATED FOOT

History

Prior to an accident in 2014, Peter Smith, then aged 51 years, had a body mass index of 29 kg/m^2 and a history of non-insulin dependent diabetes, hypertension and previous excessive alcohol intake. He had not taken alcohol for 12 years; his regular medications were metformin 2 g daily and ramipril 10 mg daily. There were several notations in the records of his general practitioner, Dr Murray Banks, that his diabetes was poorly controlled; Dr Banks had recorded no other detail about Peter's diabetes. The latest of these notations was recorded six months prior to the 2014 accident.

Peter was working at an industrial site in a subtropical city at the height of summer, when a heavy piece of metal fell onto the lateral side of his right foot. Although he was wearing safety boots, the impact of the injury was sufficient to cause lacerations to both the dorsal and the plantar surfaces of the fifth toe.

He presented to the district hospital where there was bruising and swelling in addition to the lacerations. X-rays revealed a dislocated fourth toe and a fracture of the fifth toe. The wound was cleaned, the dislocated toe was manipulated into position and he was provided with ibuprofen, paracetamol, oxycodone and amoxicillin with clavulanic acid. He was given crutches and referred to his local general practitioner for ongoing care. The hospital notes were brief, did not mention previous alcohol intake and did not include any diabetic assessment.

Peter attended Dr Banks for dressings every two days for the following month. Five days after the accident the antibiotic regimen was changed to cephalexin and metronidazole. He visited a podiatrist at the request of Dr Banks following this period of second-daily dressings to obtain advice about suitable footwear and whether he was able to return to work. The podiatrist, concerned about the state of the foot, suggested that he attend the hospital for reassessment.

The hospital notes mentioned fractures of the middle and distal phalanges of the fifth toe, the presence of diabetes and a diagnosis of osteomyelitis. At this presentation it was noted that Peter had continued with his usual diabetic medication during these three weeks. The blood glucose level on arrival at the hospital three and a half hours after food was 12.3 mmol/L (reference 5.0–8.0 mmol/L).

Peter was admitted to hospital and prescribed piperacillin and tazobactam. His diabetes was managed with frequent blood glucose measurements and short-acting insulin. When the diabetes was considered to be under control, the middle and distal phalanges of the fifth toe were amputated. Five days after the surgery he returned home on amoxicillin and clavulanic acid. The bacteriology report demonstrated the presence of pseudomonas aeruginosa, sensitive to amoxicillin and clavulanic acid. Follow-up continued at the vascular clinic of the hospital. Peter needed pregabalin for neuropathic pain for several months following the accident. He returned to his work after five months. He still needs modified footwear for work and leisure.

Legal Issues

Peter sought compensation for inadequate care following his accident, leading to the loss of his toe. The case has not yet reached a conclusion.

Discussion

A hot humid climate is an ideal environment to develop sweaty feet in a person wearing safety boots and performing hard physical work. Diabetic patients are at increased risk of fungal and bacterial infection because of likely atherosclerosis and neuropathy; they require meticulous glycaemic control and foot hygiene to minimise the risk of infection.

Staphylococcus aureus is a usual skin commensal. In diabetic patients any breach of the skin may cause staphylococcal or other infection. Peter had breaks in the skin adjacent to fractured bones; he was at high risk for osteomyelitis.

The medical record at the initial presentation to the hospital was brief. It was noted that there was a crush injury to the right fifth toe with a laceration and an underlying fracture of the fifth distal phalanx. The wound was cleaned and tetanus vaccine was administered. Although type II diabetes was mentioned, the previous history of alcohol use was not; blood glucose was not measured and there was no plan for management of diabetes. Peter was restricted to light duties for two weeks.

The junior doctor in the emergency department did not understand the danger of a compound fracture of the foot in a diabetic patient. In addition, Peter's overweight increased the risk of complications of his injury.

The emergency department doctor, by suggesting light duties for the next two weeks, showed poor understanding of work in an industrial setting. It is fortunate that Peter's employer did not allow him to go back to work initially.

Peter's assessment and management at the initial hospital presentation was inadequate. The risk for subsequent morbidity would have been reduced if an endocrinologist had been consulted to advise about optimal diabetic management.

The same comment applies to Dr Banks who had known Peter for many years. Perhaps he was complacent because of this familiarity. He was aware that Peter was overweight and had poor glycaemic control, but did not actively manage his diabetes before or after the accident.

Dr Banks' ongoing assessment was flawed. When the podiatrist saw the patient, she immediately referred him for additional assessment. Why was Dr Banks not sufficiently astute to understand that Peter needed expert care? Was this deficiency due to lack of knowledge, or was Dr Banks somehow biased because Peter was well-known to him?

At presentation to the hospital on the second occasion Peter was managed satisfactorily, including follow-up at the hospital following discharge.

Peter's major long-term problem resulting from the accident is the need for modified footwear. Unrelated to the accident is the need for both weight and diabetic control.

Dr Banks did not understand the importance of optimal glycaemic control in a diabetic patient with a potentially infected foot. He was not sufficiently clinically astute at a later time to understand that Peter needed expert help; rather the podiatrist identified this need.

The hospital managed Peter correctly at the second presentation, including the advice to Peter that ongoing care should be given at the hospital.

There is the question of the long-term outlook for Peter. It is likely that he will be able to manage with minimal disruption to his life, as the fifth toe is less important than those on the medial side of the foot.

If the metal object had fallen onto, and had broken, Peter's great toe, his level of disability would have been more severe, as that toe is of vital importance in foot stability.

Clinical Principles

There was poor assessment at the initial hospital presentation. It is always important to consider diabetic status when managing perforating injuries, especially to the lower limbs.

TYPES OF MISTAKES

We have identified a number of recurring themes in the medical negligence matters with which we have been involved over the years. The cases described in the previous chapters illustrate some of the reasons that patients sue their doctors. The medical mistakes which lead to litigation fall into three broad and overlapping categories: failure to listen and observe, failure to reason clearly and effectively, and failure to maintain appropriate professionalism. These mistakes, one way or another, amount to blind spots and roadblocks to safe medical practice.

There is no single reason for the failures of medical practice. Some reflect a lack of rigor in trying to work out the likely diagnosis for presenting complaints. Some are the result of defects in reasoning. Others are simply due to laziness, or a disregard of the fundamentals of good medical practice. Even more stem from failures to heed basic principles taught at medical schools. It may surprise many to see how obvious some of the lessons learned are, and yet time and again, there are instances where basic safeguards to prevent patient harm were not taken.

The most frequent blind spots and roadblocks we have observed are the result of not obeying one or more of the following rules (in no particular order):

1. A patient who presents with multiple symptoms usually has one diagnosis to explain the symptoms (Occam's razor).
2. If you listen carefully, a patient will usually lead you to the correct diagnosis (listen carefully).
3. A parent is often more able than a doctor to tell when his or her infant is unwell (listen to parents).
4. Always exclude organic pathology before resting on a psychiatric diagnosis (diligence).
5. Always exclude sinister pathology before accepting a benign explanation (diligence).
6. Avoid shortcuts, to reduce the risk of making diagnostic mistakes (diligence).
7. Pharmaceuticals have unwanted side effects (as do illicit drugs). Consider this whenever a prescription is written, or a patient presents with otherwise unexplained symptoms (remember drug side effects).
8. Make a sufficient list of differential diagnoses (think).
9. Common things occur commonly (think).
10. Correlate investigations to the symptoms and signs (think).
11. Keep an open mind (think).

12. When in doubt seek help from a professional colleague (ask).
13. Keep up-to-date with the literature relevant to your practice (read and review).
14. Make sure there is reliable science behind any new technology or treatment offered to a patient (read and review).
15. Ensure continuity of care (think ahead).
16. Communicate effectively with other practitioners (talk).
17. Know your limits (insight).
18. A boundary must be kept between a doctor and a patient (professionalism).
19. If concerned about a patient's condition or treatment, seek help regardless of whether this may be personally embarrassing or contrary to another doctor's views (advocate).
20. Guidelines are useful tools for diagnosis and treatment, but they are not substitutes for exercising one's own clinical judgment (think).

Occam's Razor

As we have seen, many errors resulting in litigation are more about a failure in the reasoning process of the doctor rather than deficiencies in knowledge. Diagnosis is much more about thinking and reasoning than it is about ticking off from a textbook a list of symptoms and signs associated with a particular disease. An appreciation of classic literature is probably a useful attribute when solving clinical problems.

Occam's razor is a probabilistic method of reasoning that was introduced in the fourteenth century. It is much more likely that there will be a single, unifying diagnosis rather than a number of unrelated or independent conditions to explain a patient's presenting complaints. The failure to think in this commonsense way has occasionally resulted in serious injury. It presents an impediment to accurate and prompt diagnosis.

In Steve Coates' case (Unexplained weight loss), Dr Fairweather was confronted by a history of weight loss, anxiety and altered bowel habit. Rather than thinking of a unifying diagnosis, he attributed Steve's anxiety to relationship and financial concerns, his weight loss to football training and the bowel symptoms to an infection.

All of Steve's problems were caused by a rectal carcinoma that was never diagnosed while Steve was under the care of Dr Fairweather. Ironically, Steve gave Dr Fairweather a clue about the possible diagnosis when he pointedly asked whether he had cancer. The possibility of cancer was clearly of concern. The anxiety was linked to the weight loss and blood and mucus in the bowel motions, and had little to do with relationship or other issues.

Not all of the doctors caring for John Wivell (Steroid toxicity) counselled him that his work environment was likely to have aggravated his dermatitis and conjunctivitis. With the exception of John's second general practitioner, each of the doctors he saw focused on the particular ailment with which they were presented, without considering the bigger picture of John's problems and his work. The history pointed to a common cause for his complaints, but recognition of this fact came far too late.

In Sebastian Lopez's case (Obesity), a single diagnosis was available to explain multiple ailments. Sebastian was morbidly obese. This was responsible for his diabetes, osteoarthritis, obstructive sleep apnoea and difficulty breathing. When liver function abnormalities were identified, the probability was that they were also associated with his obesity, and were not due to heavy metal toxicity in the workplace. The connection was not made; as a result, there was a delay in referring Sebastian to a hepatologist.

Barry Grant (Neck pain) presented with a fever, sore throat and neck pain. Staff in the emergency department at the hospital diagnosed him with musculoskeletal pain and a sore throat. If they had paid attention to the history of a recent laceration to the foot, and applied Occam's Razor to their reasoning, they would have thought of the possibility that there was a single diagnosis explaining all symptoms and signs. Barry's spinal epidural abscess may have been diagnosed earlier.

LISTENING AND LEARNING

Listen Carefully

Even the most inarticulate person will, if given time, and if approached in a considerate and compassionate manner, point an attentive doctor in the direction of the diagnosis. In many cases that we have seen, there has been a failure to attach significance to symptoms conveyed by a patient, together with a failure to interrogate in a targeted and focused way.

The approach to pain as a presenting symptom is often a problem. Many doctors fail to ask about time of onset, mode of onset, aggravating and relieving factors, site, radiation, etc. We frequently see cases, such as that of Krystyna Horvat (Chest pain), where ischaemic heart disease was not diagnosed simply because a proper history was not taken or understood. If Dr Jennings had listened more carefully she would have realised that Krystyna needed further investigation of ischaemic heart disease.

History taking is fundamental to clinical assessment. Students are taught systems of enquiry to help them minimise the risk that important facts might be overlooked. Practising doctors then utilise selected elements of these systems in different clinical situations. When shortcuts are taken, important features may be missed. Once missed, the gap tends to persist, as medical practitioners often rely on the initial history taken at the primary care level of general practice, or at the coalface of a hospital emergency department, when formulating a management plan. A failure to listen is a substantial impediment to safe practice.

Dr Williams failed to suspect pulmonary embolism when Gregory Merton (Haemoptysis) presented with haemoptysis after long-haul flights. If Dr Williams had listened carefully to the history, earlier diagnosis of DVT and pulmonary embolism would be likely to have occurred, and Gregory would have survived.

In the case of the lacerated foot, Peter Smith (Lacerated foot) had poorly controlled diabetes, which proved to be a significant factor in his complicated recovery. The doctor initially treated the laceration and bony injuries, but failed to listen carefully to Peter's medical history. He then failed to recognise that management of diabetes was just as important as primary wound care. Fortunately, Peter's loss of his small toe had little functional significance, but it may have been worse.

Tom Wood's (Sore wrist) wrist was injured in a motor vehicle accident. A scaphoid fracture was seen on x-ray, but was not acted upon. This history was overlooked when he presented later with a thumb injury, and it was only after consultations with several specialists that the scaphoid fracture was finally addressed. If the various general practitioners and orthopaedic consultants had taken more time to listen carefully to the history, Tom's outcome in relation to his wrist may have been better.

Amanda Gordon's death (Postnatal depression) by suicide may not have occurred if proper attention had been given to her story. Early after giving birth to her son, Amanda described anxiety, panic, insomnia and a low mood. She also expressed thoughts of self-harm, and even attempted to end her life by taking an overdose of oxazepam. Once she was admitted to hospital, she explicitly referred to a plan of suicide by driving herself into the wilderness.

The night before her death Amanda attempted to explain to staff that she was fearful of going on leave, and that she had dark thoughts including suicidal ideation when away from the hospital. This history should have rung very loud alarm bells to the psychiatric staff. They failed to hear what Amanda was saying to them. As a result, she was given unrestricted leave and committed suicide.

LISTEN TO PARENTS

An infant cannot provide any verbal history. An older child may not be able to give a coherent history because of undeveloped language skills. Therefore, medical practitioners must rely on parents or other adult family members to obtain a history. Parents will know how a child behaves normally, and will certainly know when a child is seriously unwell. Of course, there will always be the anxious parent who takes a child to a doctor for minor ailments, but when it comes to serious illnesses, a doctor would be foolhardy to ignore the concerns of a parent and any history they give of significant change in behaviour.

By not listening carefully to a parent, who can be assumed to have intimate knowledge of the child's condition, a doctor places too much reliance on physical examination, and deprives him or herself of a valuable source of information.

Margaret Buchanan challenged Dr Crowhurst's diagnosis of tonsillitis when Maddie (Ingestion of a caustic solution) had symptoms suggesting ingestion of a caustic substance and not suggesting tonsillitis. Dr Crowhurst persisted with her original wrong diagnosis at review a week later. If Dr Crowhurst had been less rigid in her thinking and had been prepared to admit she was wrong, Maddie's oesophageal damage would have been recognised and managed sooner, likely with a better outcome for Maddie.

Morag Maclean (Mother knows best) knew that Aiden was unwell. If Dr Hunter had thoroughly considered everything that Morag told him about Aiden's illness endocarditis would have been discovered sooner, antibiotic therapy would have been commenced earlier and aortic valve replacement may have been avoided.

Kylie Miller's (A sick infant) acute appendicitis may have been diagnosed sooner if Dr Holmes had given more weight to her mother's concerns about her daughter.

Diligence

Always exclude organic pathology

Two of the most common blind spots we have seen concern failures to think the worst when patients present with unusual or repetitive complaints. While it may be easy to diagnose a cold or a broken leg, thinking more widely seems to be a problem for many doctors. This may be a function of the time available to see a patient in a busy practice, laziness or a failure to listen carefully to the patient. It is unlikely to be due to stupidity.

Shortly after she gave birth to her daughter, Ruby Chen (Delirium) suffered an episode of acute delirium. Because of a prior history of drug and alcohol abuse, staff were suspicious of a form of intoxication, including an overdose of benzodiazepines smuggled into the hospital.

Although a CT brain scan was ordered to screen for non-psychiatric causes for the delirium, this was at best a half-hearted attempt to exclude organic pathology. If medical staff were serious about excluding an organic cause, including an infection, then an MRI scan of the brain should have been ordered. If an organic cause had been properly investigated, then Ruby's cryptococcal meningitis would have been diagnosed earlier. She would have been treated earlier and had a better long-term outcome.

Always exclude sinister pathology

There are certain symptoms that should cause alarm bells to ring for all doctors, but particularly those in general practice or in emergency departments. Such symptoms include complaints like unexplained weight loss, bleeding from the rectum, haemoptysis after long-haul air travel, etc. While many of these symptoms or signs may have potentially benign causes, they may also be associated with serious, life-threatening conditions. In these circumstances, a doctor should be dogged in first excluding a sinister cause before resting comfortably on a more benign explanation for the complaints. We have found that this frequently does not occur.

As mentioned above, Dr Crowhurst (Ingestion of a caustic solution) diagnosed tonsillitis in Maddie Buchanan, without seriously considering or excluding ingestion of a caustic substance.

Dr Cunningham thought about the possibility of sinister tongue pathology in Deepak Sharma's case (Tongue cancer), but thought a nonspecific CT scan of the neck was sufficient to exclude it. If a practitioner thinks sinister pathology is possible, then full investigation must be completed. There is no point in taking half measures.

Dr Ewart and Mr Lucas both failed to exclude DVT when Suzana Lazarevic (Mechanism of stroke) had acute onset calf pain after immobilisation of the leg following fracture. DVT and thromboembolism via a PFO may have caused Suzana's subsequent stroke. If DVT had been suspected and confirmed, Suzana would have received anticoagulation and stroke may have been avoided.

Dr Subahdar, a cardiologist, rejected the provisional diagnosis of endocarditis in his patient Dawn Norville (Persistently unwell) on the basis of a normal CRP. He then failed to notice that the CRP had risen, and did not offer any diagnosis other than endocarditis. He declined to look after his patient, who was admitted to hospital under the care of a gastroenterologist. Dawn's prosthetic valve endocarditis was treated too late and she died.

Steve Coates (Unexplained weight loss) presented to his general practitioner and Dr Fairweather with two alarming problems: rectal bleeding, and excessive unexplained weight loss. These factors should have been red flags to Dr Fairweather about the potential for colorectal cancer and the need for colonoscopy. This did not occur until it was too late to save Steve's life.

In Willem Amundsen's case (Syncope), syncope was attributed to a vasovagal response without first excluding more sinister possibilities, such as long QT syndrome.

Baby Damian (Toxoplasmosis) was born with congenital heart disease and unrelated hepatomegaly. He was seen by numerous general practitioners over several years before being referred to a paediatrician who diagnosed toxoplasmosis. By then Damian was severely and permanently disabled by a disease which could have been treated years before. Had any of the doctors involved in the care of Damian soon after birth considered serious treatable causes of hepatomegaly, Damian may have enjoyed a better outcome.

No shortcuts to making the correct diagnosis

It appears obvious that a thorough history and examination are required in order to deliver a rational list of differential diagnoses and to make a provisional diagnosis. It is staggering how many times this general rule is broken.

Many doctors may take short cuts. Nine times out of ten they might get away with them. But ultimately, bad practice has a habit of catching up with them.

Dr Tan would likely have diagnosed Boris Umanoff's penile cancer (Penile cancer) when Boris first presented to him if Dr Tan had taken an adequate history. When the penile lesion grew following application of podophyllotoxin cream, Dr Tan persevered with his incorrect diagnosis of "wart on penis". If Dr Tan had been prepared to question his first diagnosis when Boris's symptoms failed to resolve, biopsy would likely have revealed cancer which could have been treated earlier than was the case, perhaps with a better outcome.

Barry Grant's spinal epidural abscess (Neck pain) would likely have been diagnosed much sooner if there had been attention given to his past history of illicit drug use and his elevated temperature.

Physical examination is as integral to clinical assessment as is proper history taking. Unfortunately, many of the cases we have discussed involved only cursory examinations, or no examinations at all.

Dr Fairweather failed to perform a rectal examination on Steve Coates (Unexplained weight loss). This ultimately meant that his rectal cancer was diagnosed late in its course. It is likely to have been curable if time had been taken by Dr Fairweather to perform a comprehensive examination.

Dr Williams failed to examine Gregory Merton's calves (Haemoptysis). If he had, he may well have detected signs of DVT. This would have led to proper investigation, diagnosis of thrombosis and treatment that would have avoided pulmonary embolism and death.

Shirley Finney (Shoulder pain) was an ex-drug addict with lupus erythematosus, who presented with neurological symptoms, and evidence of infection. She was reviewed by numerous doctors who did not perform a neurological examination, resulting in delayed care, and permanent quadriplegia.

Elizabeth Paskin (Sagging lip) had transient neurological symptoms and signs. She was not referred for immediate assessment in hospital, and suffered a debilitating stroke, which may have been prevented, or the effects reduced, if she had been referred to hospital when she first presented. In this case, Dr Surubian did not appear to understand basic neuroanatomy; she performed an inadequate examination and was unable to synthesise appropriate differential diagnoses based on history and physical examination.

Tom Wood (Sore wrist) had attended his general practitioner with wrist pain on several occasions over four months with stitches still in situ. The stitches of themselves were not the problem. The failure to examine the wrist was a manifestation of inadequate assessment generally; too many shortcuts were taken. If the wrist had been examined systematically, scaphoid tenderness would likely have been detected and the outcome improved.

Kylie Miller (A sick infant) was not examined when she first presented with abdominal pain and vomiting. Dr Holmes took shortcuts. If the abdomen had been examined for tenderness and rebound, and if the temperature had been recorded, important signs of appendicitis would likely have been elicited earlier than was the case, and she would not likely have suffered life threatening peritonitis with the prospect of widespread intraabdominal adhesions and a risk of bowel obstruction in the future.

Stan Crockett's spinal cord tumour (Leg weakness) may have been diagnosed earlier if Dr Ahmed had been more diligent in reading the clinical records prior to his consultation. He would have realised that only a CT scan of the spine had been performed. His management of Mr Crockett's condition was based upon the false assumption that an MRI scan had already been ordered. This led him to diagnose a rare polyneuropathy. Reasonable diligence would have alerted Dr Ahmed earlier to his mistake.

Diligence extends to thorough investigation of particular complaints. Doctors Valentine, Carmichael, Gonzales and Goldblatt all failed to thoroughly investigate breast lumps in their patients (Breast lumps). They ignored the guidelines that were available to help them. Dr Ongley

(Visual disturbance) failed to exclude cardiac causes of recurrent transient neurological deficits.

Remember drug side effects

Both prescription and illicit drugs have side effects that may influence a patient's presentation or explain unusual symptoms or signs.

The case of Trudy Mawson (A pharmacological nightmare) illustrated a plethora of drug effects. Dr O'Toole and Mr Gladstone failed to appreciate the risk of precipitating with drugs a lethal ventricular arrhythmia in a patient with QT prolongation. Barry Grant (Neck pain) had a history of intravenous drug use, which put him at an increased risk of infection. When he presented to the emergency department with a fever and neck pain, an infective cause should have been considered. Staff in the emergency department failed to attach any significance to the history of drug use.

John Wivell's steroid-induced glaucoma (Steroid toxicity) could have been avoided if his multiple medical practitioners had remembered that drugs have potential side effects.

Beryl Austin (Headache) received an overdose of heparin and experienced generalised bleeding. The risk of a life-threatening side effect of heparin, intracerebral haemorrhage, was not recognised until it was too late.

Professor Harrington (Childhood cancer) did not appreciate the risk of potentially debilitating side effects of intrathecal chemotherapy in conjunction with radiotherapy to the spine.

THINKING AND REASONING

Differential Diagnoses

Many of the maxims of medicine are interrelated. One reflection of inadequate reasoning is the frequent failure of medical practitioners to consider a list of reasonably available differential diagnoses. Medical students are taught to be alert for potentially serious diagnoses to explain clinical features, rather than to make a presumptive diagnosis of a benign condition. Common and uncommon causes need to be evaluated in turn.

Emergency staff assessing Barry Grant (Neck pain) assumed that he had neck pain of benign musculoskeletal origin rather than considering a proper list of differential diagnoses, which should have included spinal cord pathology in general, and infection in particular. If they had done so, then a proper investigation by way of an MRI scan of the spine would have been performed and his quadriplegia avoided.

In Steve Coates' case (Unexplained weight loss), Dr Fairweather, although pondering the need for a colonoscopy (which was never performed), failed to have colorectal cancer on his radar. Given Steve's presentation with unexplained weight loss, and blood and mucus in his bowel motions, colorectal cancer should have been high on a list of differential diagnoses. Dr Fairweather never organised his thoughts sufficiently to create such a list.

Amanda Gordon (Postnatal depression) was managed for postpartum depression and insomnia, but her risk of suicide was ignored and she was allowed to go on unescorted leave. If the risk of suicide had been acknowledged, and if she had remained supervised, she would likely have lived.

Kylie Miller (A sick infant) was initially diagnosed with constipation when she presented with abdominal pain and vomiting due to appendicitis. Dr Holmes developed a list of differential diagnoses including constipation and gastroenteritis, but never included acute appendicitis on the list. He did not record Kylie's temperature or note whether there was any localised abdominal pain or rebound tenderness. The diagnosis may not have been considered because Kylie was only two years of age, but Dr Holmes did not even seriously entertain the possibility of other forms of bowel pathology.

Likewise, Josh Medhurst's acute appendicitis and rupture (An avoidable tragedy) was not appreciated promptly because Dr Feeney thought he had bowel obstruction and failed to consider the potential causes of the obstruction.

Willem Amundsen (Syncope) had a history of syncope and his mother had symptoms (which may have been due to self-terminating torsades de pointes), which had been attributed to temporal lobe epilepsy. Willem was assessed by a paediatric neurologist, who concluded that he did not have epilepsy. A differential diagnosis of cardiac syncope was not even considered. It seemed that once epilepsy had been excluded, all practitioners assumed that his syncopal episodes were simply vasovagal, even though the circumstances of his presentations invited other explanations. Willem subsequently had presyncope and syncope. It was only after he had a brain injury due to ventricular fibrillation that long QT syndrome was considered.

Maria Stavros (Visual disturbance) had recurrent neurological symptoms and an atrial septal aneurysm. Although it was originally planned to perform a transoesophageal echocardiogram to exclude a PFO, this investigation was only performed after Maria had a disabling stroke associated with her atrial septal aneurysm and PFO. Her stroke may well have been prevented if the potentially lethal combination of atrial septal aneurysm and PFO had been properly diagnosed when she presented with recurrent neurological symptoms.

Skye Bannister (Dyspnoea) had dyspnoea and chest pain. A diagnosis of pleurodynia was made in the absence of fever, malaise, abdominal pain and headache. No serious alternative diagnoses were considered.

Gregory Merton's (Haemoptysis) haemoptysis after long-haul air travel was not even considered as being due to pulmonary embolism.

Krystyna Horvat (Chest pain) had recurrent exertional chest pain. For whatever reason, Dr Jennings formed the opinion that Krystyna did not have ischaemic heart disease. Symptoms of myocardial ischaemia were consequently ignored and she died of an acute myocardial infarction.

Terry Gammell (Unexplained fever) was unwell with rigors following dental work. When he presented with wrist pain due to embolism of infected material from the mitral valve, a diagnosis of endocarditis was not considered. It was only after he had an embolic stroke that appropriate investigations to confirm or exclude bacterial endocarditis were made.

Doctors Cox and Ahmed did not consider that Stan Crockett (Leg weakness) had spinal cord pathology; in consequence, potentially disability-limiting surgery was delayed.

If a medical practitioner does not create a list of differential diagnoses, then the route to accurate diagnosis is compromised. A failure to think of alternative diagnoses is a serious road block to safe medical practice.

Common Things Occur Commonly

At first glance, this dictum might appear inconsistent with the rule that sinister pathology needs to be excluded before making a diagnosis of a benign condition. It may also appear incompatible with the rule that a psychiatric diagnosis should only be made after organic pathology has been excluded. It is in fact the other side of the same coin.

Too often, a medical practitioner ignores a common condition and chases rare possibilities down multiple diagnostic holes. This may lead to a delay in diagnosis and a poor outcome for the patient. If a realistic list of differential diagnoses was entertained at the outset, then presumably common causes would be considered along with rare but potentially devastating conditions.

Dr Ahmed, for example, was convinced that Stan Crockett (Leg weakness) suffered from a rare polyneuropathy when a central nervous system problem was much more likely and needed to be excluded by an MRI scan as one of the first steps in the diagnostic work up.

Correlate Investigations to the Symptoms and Signs

Many practitioners treat investigations, particularly imaging, as a means of diagnosis in isolation. Accurate diagnoses must always entail correlating the symptoms, signs and results of investigations.

Maria Stavros (Visual disturbance) reported neurological symptoms to her general practitioner husband, who promptly referred her to appropriate specialists. The histories recorded by the different doctors varied one from one another. While this of itself is not unusual or wrong, the important error was that the subjective symptoms were conflated with unrelated imaging changes. The imaging changes were dismissed as benign and the causes of the symptoms were ignored. If the symptoms had been pursued with proper attention to the detail of the history, Maria's major stroke would have been avoided.

Jade Byrne (A number of health concerns) had a number of health concerns including exertional angina pectoris. There was suboptimal imaging at coronary angiography. Despite clear evidence to the contrary, Dr Yong concluded that Jade's arteries were normal and Jade was not treated for ischaemic heart disease. Dr Yong's error influenced the interpretation of Jade's symptoms by others. The subsequent diagnosis and management of myocardial infarction was delayed because it was believed that Jade had normal arteries. If Dr Yong had correlated Jade's symptoms with the angiographic findings, Jade may have avoided permanent left ventricular dysfunction and physical disability.

Dr Cox failed to realise that an MRI scan had not been performed of Stan Crockett's spinal cord (Leg weakness). He deprived himself of an important piece of information which, if combined with Stan's presenting symptoms and signs, would have led to a diagnosis of spinal cord tumour.

Dr Gonzales knew that Linda Forrest (Breast lumps) had a breast lump, and she knew that two different imaging modalities had detected abnormalities. Yet she did not correlate all these findings to conclude that biopsy was required (biopsy was indicated anyway according to contemporary guidelines for investigation of breast lumps).

Hayley Campbell (Cerebral palsy) suffered cerebral palsy due to an hypoxic-ischaemic insult during labour. Nursing and obstetric staff failed to appreciate that the fetal heart rate was abnormal, and mandated emergency delivery. Cardiotocography is performed for a purpose. It is used to provide early evidence of fetal distress; the staff should have realised that the heart rhythm abnormalities were related to augmentation of labour with oxytocin.

At her initial presentation, Skye Bannister (Dyspnoea) had poor R-wave progression and low voltage QRS complexes, likely due to cardiomyopathy. Right axis deviation was likely due to previous pulmonary embolism. If these abnormalities had been identified and investigated further, it is probable that cardiomyopathy and pulmonary embolism would have been diagnosed sooner than was the case.

Dr Liu knew that Lydia Milton (Palpitations) had benign ectopic beats that did not interfere with her life. Lydia told him that flecainide had made her unwell. Nevertheless Dr Liu suggested an electrophysiological study without first stopping flecainide to see if Lydia would feel better without "treatment". Dr Liu was not obliged to perform an electrophysiological procedure just because he could. Lydia required a prosthetic aortic valve as a result of a complication of Dr Liu's procedure.

In Tom Wood's case (Sore wrist), an undisplaced scaphoid fracture was reported on an x-ray, but this was never correlated with any clinical signs or symptoms. Tom had in fact complained to Dr Taniane of pain at the site of the scaphoid fracture. If the significance of the localised pain and the x-ray findings had not been overlooked, he might have had a better outcome.

Harry Adams (Rectal bleeding) had cancer demonstrated on histopathology of a rectal polyp. The polyp was snared, but appropriate surveillance was not arranged. If the significance of the histological diagnosis had been recognised, follow-up would have been closer, and he may not have died of cancer.

Krystyna Horvat (Chest pain) had classical symptoms of myocardial ischaemia in the context of a family history of ischaemic heart disease and diabetes mellitus, and a personal history of cigarette smoking, obesity, hypertension and hypercholesterolaemia. The absence of reversible ischaemia on a stress echocardiogram did not exclude the presence of atherosclerotic ischaemic heart disease. A negative result for the stress echocardiogram could not be viewed in isolation from the history and symptoms of chest pain. Further investigation was required because the negative result did not correlate with the clinical presentation. The findings of a subsequent stress echocardiogram, which suggested myocardial ischaemia, were not recognised by the cardiologist or reported to the general practitioner.

Lucy Simpson (Missed period) had an ectopic pregnancy and was fortunate not to bleed to death. She had clinical and biochemical evidence of pregnancy and an empty uterus. The diagnosis of ectopic pregnancy was not considered until it was nearly too late. Simple correlation of investigation results with her presentation should have led to an earlier diagnosis.

Dr Garcia (Obesity) did not appreciate that abnormal LFTs could be caused by obesity. This led to a failure to manage the obesity effectively and increased the risk that Sebastian would die of liver cancer.

Keep an Open Mind

Many of the errors we have identified may be due to inflexible thinking. Very often, doctors make a diagnosis and then for whatever reason are reluctant to discard that diagnosis, and think that a patient's symptoms and signs may be due to another condition. Entrenchment of a diagnosis can be harmful and, on occasions, fatal to a patient.

Dr Geraty accepted the history related by Anne Kirkup (Family dynamics) about her father's behaviour. Dr Geraty did not question the second-hand diagnosis of paranoia, and inappropriately arranged involuntary admission of Rohan to a psychiatric facility.

Alice Tunbridge (Things may not be as they seem) attended numerous doctors at a general practice clinic and feigned illnesses that she did not have. She was addicted to narcotics. Towards the end of her life, one of Alice's doctors suspected Munchausen syndrome but did not pursue the diagnosis. No one sought to request medical records from the hospital to which Alice said she had been admitted.

Dr Cunningham, an ENT surgeon, examined Deepak Sharma (Tongue cancer) because of right-sided ear ache. In the absence of evidence of another diagnosis Dr Cunningham diagnosed middle ear infection, for which he prescribed antibiotics. Deepak's symptoms persisted, and the next year Dr Cunningham requested a CT scan as a screen for cancer, but did not take his investigations any further. Deepak then consulted Dr Smith, a neurologist, who investigated further and diagnosed malignancy in the tongue, for which Deepak underwent glossectomy by Dr Franklin. If Dr Cunningham had been more assiduous in his diagnostic approach when Deepak had persistent symptoms despite therapy, cancer would likely have been diagnosed sooner and Deepak may not have lost his entire tongue.

Dr Jennings probably formed a first impression that Krystyna Horvat (Chest pain) did not have ischaemic heart disease (without careful consideration of all the evidence to the contrary). Having established this thought, Dr Jennings failed to reconsider the possibility of ischaemic heart disease. Her mind was not sufficiently open to consider that her first impression may have been wrong. A doctor should be prepared to retake a history when a diagnosis appears to be wrong, or if expected improvement does not occur.

In Sebastian Lopez's case (Obesity) Dr Garcia did not connect the abnormal LFTs with Sebastian's obesity. He thought the obesity was a separate problem and the liver function abnormalities were due to workplace exposure to toxins. If he had reviewed his diagnoses earlier, then Sebastian may have been referred to a hepatologist earlier.

When Dr Holmes diagnosed Kylie Miller (A sick infant) with constipation, he simply did not consider appendicitis as a possibility. Even when a colleague made the correct diagnosis of appendicitis Dr Holmes dismissed the possibility. Closed-mindedness probably inhibited Dr Holmes' physical examination and interpretation of findings. If he had a more open mind, he would likely have examined Kylie more thoroughly, and considered a range of diagnostic possibilities.

In many of the cases we have discussed, differential diagnoses simply were not made, or were discarded without sufficient consideration. Thoughtful practitioners develop techniques to reduce the risk of being closed-minded. Some may write down diagnostic possibilities as they come to mind, so that they are not forgotten later during the consultation. Others may actively consider alternatives to an initial provisional diagnosis in order not to overlook an important alternative diagnosis.

Shirley Finney (Shoulder pain) presented at a teaching hospital with shoulder pain. A hospital doctor noted that she was ataxic, but performed no neurologic examination. She then had sensations like electric shocks in her arm and was treated with sedation and antidepressant therapy by Dr Sokolov.

Dr Sokolov was not sufficiently open-minded to consider that ataxia and paraesthesia may have a common origin. It is probable that failure to have an open mind influenced the hospital doctor who next examined Shirley. Whatever the actual physical findings were, the hospital doctor did not take account of the previous history, and diagnosed ataxia following a seizure, although Shirley had not had a fit. If more time had been taken to thoughtfully consider all the preceding symptoms, without being influenced by previously wrong diagnoses, then earlier investigation would likely have led to a better outcome.

Sometimes a doctor makes a correct diagnosis, only to be dissuaded from it thereafter. Dr Goldblatt discovered Miriam Irving's breast lump and enlarged axillary lymph nodes (Breast lumps), and arranged an ultrasound. When the imaging did not confirm his suspicion of cancer, he closed his mind to the possibility and failed to proceed with a biopsy, thereby delaying the diagnosis of cancer.

GUIDELINES

We have noticed a recent and increasing trend for doctors to be asked to adhere to guidelines or protocols when diagnosing or managing patients. We have concerns about this development.

There is no question that guidelines can assist in the diagnostic process. Diagnostic and treatment algorithms exist for many common emergency conditions such as chest pain or stroke. These are useful tools so long as medical practitioners understand that blind adherence to the protocols may not always be in a patient's best interest. Sometimes, it is necessary to think outside the box so as to ensure that a serious diagnosis is not missed.

The same applies to treatment guidelines. While many guidelines may be based on reputable epidemiological studies, they may not be relevant to individual cases where management must be tailored based on clinical judgment. Medical practitioners are trained and skilled professionals. We don't think that compelling them to follow guidelines will reduce litigation. Despite this view, we anticipate that the trend will continue.

Dawn Norville (Persistently unwell) may have survived if Dr Subahdar had not excluded prosthetic endocarditis in purported reliance on the Duke criteria.

Josh Medhurst (An avoidable tragedy) probably would be alive today if he had been first taken to a tertiary hospital offering paediatric surgical facilities rather than to the nearest hospital with a paediatric ward in accordance with emergency protocols.

PROFESSIONALISM AND INSIGHT

Ask

Hayley Campbell's cerebral palsy (Cerebral palsy) was caused by a failure to recognise the nonreassuring fetal heart rate pattern as well as inappropriate use of oxytocin. Senior obstetric staff were not called in to assess Grace's labour with her daughter. There was a deficiency in knowledge and education, leading to the staff not recognising the significance of the abnormal fetal heart rate pattern.

The fact that the heart rhythm normalised when oxytocin was suspended should have prompted early consultation with senior colleagues. The junior obstetric staff needed to recognise the limits of their expertise and call in the consultant obstetrician for advice. The outcome may well have been different if this had occurred.

Liz Chadwick (Abdominal pain) had a biliary leak because Dr Briggs did not ask for help when he encountered difficulty securing the common bile duct. Dr Holmes actively avoided accepting help in sorting out Kylie Miller's abdominal pain. Dr Harland did not ask for help when confronted with evidence of pregnancy, but an empty uterus. Professor Harrington did not ask for advice about therapy, even though others at his hospital were more up-to-date than he was.

Doctors Curnow, Penklis, Mweratua and Halloran all failed to consider a diagnosis of cauda equina syndrome (Cauda equina syndrome), and failed to recognise that the symptoms reported by their patients mandated immediate neurosurgical review. This may have been due to a fundamental lack of knowledge of neuroanatomy, or it may have been due to a reluctance to seek advice from others.

Since one cannot know what one doesn't know, it is important to be aware of this fact and to actively seek advice when symptoms and signs do not match a recognised diagnosis. Always consider and exclude a potentially serious differential diagnosis before settling on a benign diagnosis. It is often necessary to obtain the advice of others to satisfy this principle.

Read and Review

Keep up-to-date

Medical school education aims to provide a broad knowledge base upon which medical graduates can build throughout their working lives. Entrance to some medical schools requires aptitude assessment, to identify those individuals most likely to become "good doctors". Some medical schools require successful completion of a previous undergraduate degree, to encourage a broader education than is possible in a program focused entirely on medical science.

The assessment and examination processes at university are designed to ensure that medical graduates are adequately equipped to develop as effective and safe clinicians. Medical education, however, has finite physical, financial and human resources. It is impossible to guarantee that every graduate has the knowledge to address every clinical challenge. Ultimately, each doctor is personally responsible to review their knowledge and practice habits, and to keep up-to-date with contemporary standards in their relevant area of practice.

In order to maintain medical registration, it is necessary to satisfy certain minimum continuing professional development (CPD) criteria. All professional colleges maintain CPD programs. These colleges also provide, and update, guidelines for management of various illnesses. Scientific meetings and conferences are held frequently. There can be no excuse for practitioners not being across the scientific literature relevant to management of patients in their particular area of practice.

Doctors O'Mara, Brown and Crawford (Necrotising fasciitis) all failed to consider at first the possibility of potentially fatal necrotising fasciitis. Barbara Napaljarri lost her life; Beryl Dooley lost her breasts; and Brian Schipp had a gangrenous scrotum. All these complications may have been avoided with early suspicion of the diagnosis and early intravenous antibiotic therapy.

Dr Garcia (Obesity) ran into a roadblock through lack of knowledge when he failed to recognise the connection between Sebastian's morbid obesity and his chronic liver dysfunction.

Mary Kilpatrick (Childhood cancer) suffered the devastating consequences of transverse myelitis because she received outmoded chemotherapy for the treatment of her soft tissue sarcoma. If Professor Harrington had kept abreast of the relevant literature for the treatment of her tumour, she would not have received intrathecal chemotherapy and certainly would not have received such therapy concurrently with radiation therapy. Her quadriplegia would have been avoided.

The cases of breast cancer (Breast lumps) illustrate the need to keep up-to-date with contemporary guidelines. The principle of triple testing was established in 1997, but was ignored by Doctors Valentine, Carmichael, Gonzales and Goldblatt when investigating their patients with breast lumps.

New technology

In many ways, this is an extension of the obligation to keep up-to-date more generally. Medical practitioners are frequently asked, or encouraged, to take up new treatments, whether it be new devices or new pharmaceuticals. Not all new treatments are rigorously tested by way of randomised controlled trials (RCTs) before they are introduced to the market. For example, class II medical devices may be entered on the Australian Register of

Therapeutic Goods (ARTG) without the manufacturer having completed any RCT to satisfy the long-term safety and efficacy of the product. Recent public examples have been the metal-on-metal hip replacement system manufactured by DePuy and the transvaginal mesh kits manufactured by Ethicon.

These devices were entered onto the ARTG because they were found to have substantial equivalence to previous devices. This means that, if a device is deemed to be similar to an existing device, there is no need for RCTs or other studies to prove the safety and efficacy of the new technology.

Even if a device has been validly registered with the Therapeutic Goods Administration (TGA), it is still necessary for medical practitioners to explain carefully to their patients the quality of the evidence supporting the safety and effectiveness of the treatment, to explain that not all risks are known and to give fair and unbiased information about alternative treatments. If a doctor does not recommend an alternative treatment because he or she does not use the alternative, then a second opinion might be considered so that a patient can receive information not only in relation to the new technology, but also about reasonably available alternatives.

Christine Talbot (Pelvic organ prolapse) was treated with a transvaginal mesh that caused significant pain and distress. She continues to have problems. She alleged that she was not given enough or balanced information to satisfy herself that it was in her interest to have the mesh implanted to repair her pelvic organ prolapse rather than more traditional methods. Dr Anderson might have considered he was justified in using the mesh because the TGA had registered it and, as such, he was entitled to use it. He might have thought he was justified in assuming it was safe for use because it was on the ARTG.

Sue Massey (A mesh by any other name) would have avoided life-altering pelvic pain if Dr Mulcahy had been aware of the nature of the TFS he implanted and the results of the studies concerning its safety and efficacy.

Think Ahead

Continuity of care is relevant both in multiple general practitioner medical centres, where a patient may see different doctors on different occasions, and in the context of a referring general practitioner and a specialist or hospital.

Proper continuity of care can only occur with appropriate record keeping, and sharing of data between relevant parties. If a subsequent treater cannot understand what occurred previously, and the patient may be unable to fill in the gaps, then the subsequent treater may be at risk of serious diagnostic error.

Alice Tunbridge (Things may not be as they seem) attended numerous doctors at a general practice clinic. Record keeping was inadequate and communication between the doctors about Alice's complaints was poor. If record keeping had been up to a proper standard, Munchausen syndrome may have been recognised sooner, her condition may have been managed better and Alice may not have died when she did.

Terry Gammell (Unexplained fever) saw a number of different general practitioners, none of whom took responsibility to investigate his multiple complaints to arrive at a unifying diagnosis. The diagnosis of bacterial endocarditis was missed to Terry's detriment.

Dr Briggs failed to document details of the cholecystectomy he performed on Liz Chadwick (Abdominal pain). He did not describe difficulty ligating the bile duct, and he did not recognise the bile leak thereafter. If he had admitted his difficulty during the operation, he might have sought the assistance of an experienced colleague. Ultimately, working out what happened became a forensic exercise in legal proceedings rather than something that should have been evident from the operative record.

If Dr Briggs had followed prudent practice he would have documented his operative findings accurately. He and others would then more likely have recognised earlier the bile leak. Documentation of detailed operative findings is often of benefit to subsequent carers, particularly if reoperation is required.

Dr Shadbolt requested a swab be taken from Jake Toohey (Failed hip replacement) when there was a discharge from his wound after hip replacement. The wound swab grew methicillin-sensitive Staphylococcus aureus, but Dr Shadbolt did not follow up the result. Appropriate antibiotic treatment was delayed, debridement surgery was unsuccessful, and the prosthetic hip had to be removed. If Dr Shadbolt had thought ahead and ensured that the swab result was reviewed promptly Jake would have had the chance of a better outcome.

Talk

Dr Bonnici knew that Camilla Torrington (Toxoplasmosis) may have had active toxoplasmosis in early pregnancy. The pathologist advised serial blood testing. Dr Bonnici did not pass this information on to Camilla, or to the other doctors caring for Camilla. Baby Florence was born with toxoplasmosis and was permanently disabled as a result.

Dr Philpott, a general practitioner, neglected to advise staff in the maternity ward of Alana Blum's therapy with clozapine for drug-resistant schizophrenia (Restraint). Following delivery of baby Stephen, Alana did not take her clozapine regularly, became catatonic, and was scheduled to the psychiatric unit as an involuntary patient. Alana had alternating agitation and catatonia, and auditory hallucinations. She was inadequately supervised, and ingested a caustic substance from a cleaner's trolley. She became violently distressed, was restrained in a prone position by several staff, had a cardiorespiratory arrest due to asphyxia and died 2 weeks later of ischaemic encephalopathy. If Alana's schizophrenia had been optimally treated after Stephen's birth, she would likely have survived.

The paediatric neurologist who saw Willem Amundsen (Syncope) did not talk to a cardiologist about possible cardiac causes for syncope. If he had done so, it is likely that Willem's long QT syndrome would have been discovered before he had an hypoxic brain injury.

Communication with Kylie Miller (A sick infant) was difficult because she was two years old. There was no direct communication between Dr Holmes and the after-hours locum. Dr Holmes did not consult with others to assist with diagnosing Kylie's illness. If Dr Holmes had talked to the locum rather than simply dismissing the locum's opinion, he may well have learned that appendicitis was the appropriate working diagnosis, and allowed earlier treatment.

Dr Williams and the radiologist did not discuss adequately the optimal investigations to determine the cause of Gary Merton's haemoptysis. If they had talked with each other, pulmonary embolism would likely have been diagnosed and treated effectively.

Maria Stavros saw several doctors, including her husband. None of the doctors discussed with each other their opinions or diagnostic plans. It is at least possible, and more likely probable, that if there had been thoughtful discussion between the various medical practitioners, the significance of the clinical history and investigations would have been correctly interpreted.

John Wivell was seen by numerous doctors (including general practitioners, ophthalmologists, dermatologists and an immunologist). The first dermatologist counselled Dr Roberts about the risks of potent steroids; Dr Roberts ignored the advice. Uncoordinated management, without thoughtful discussion between the various doctors, probably contributed to the long-term prescription of steroid facial creams and eye drops that caused glaucoma and visual impairment.

In an inpatient scenario, medical practitioners should remember that nursing staff spend more hours in contact with patients than they do. Accordingly, nursing staff may have an important advantage in understanding the mental state and physical condition of patients. Doctors should attach significance to communications made to them by nursing staff. Of course, nursing staff should likewise recognise the importance of their own professional input. For instance, if Amanda Gordon's disturbing history of anxiety and suicidal ideation had been communicated to hospital psychiatrists, she would probably not have been granted unescorted leave and would not likely have committed suicide when she did.

Advocate

A medical practitioner, particularly a general practitioner, should be an advocate for his or her patients. There are likely to be many occasions when a doctor will doubt the prudence of proposed or instituted treatment, or question the accuracy or reasonableness of a diagnosis. It is generally appropriate to rely on the views of the most experienced, skilled or knowledgeable practitioner. But this does not mean a less experienced or specialised doctor can altogether abrogate responsibility. Often, general practitioners know more about a patient than a specialist because the therapeutic relationship has existed for longer. Junior doctors in a public hospital setting may have spent more time going over a history at presentation. There is nothing wrong with asking for a second opinion or querying current management. Such queries should ideally be met with proper professional courtesy. Many junior doctors or general practitioners may feel awkward about imposing on a senior or specialist colleague. They may in consequence not take steps that are in their patients' interests. There is no place in the practice of medicine for personal embarrassment, anxiety or silence to compromise proper care.

When Margaret Buchanan's parents took Maddie (Ingestion of a caustic solution) to the local emergency department Maddie was appropriately seen by a senior emergency medicine specialist and a consultant paediatrician. A differential diagnosis to be excluded was ingestion of a caustic substance. Review at the tertiary children's hospital was not as appropriate. Whereas the junior emergency medical staff understood that caustic ingestion was to be excluded, the ENT registrar thought otherwise and no senior specialist was consulted. If the junior staff had not felt obliged to defer to the opinion of the ENT registrar, and had access to senior specialists, it is likely that the correct diagnosis would have been secured sooner than it was.

Dr Donoghue arranged a second trimester ultrasound for Pamela McNamara (An obstetric abnormality). The radiologist observed high risk features on the scan and phoned Dr Donoghue. Dr Donoghue either failed to grasp the significance of the scan findings, or simply chose not to consult immediately with the obstetrician. Earlier consultant obstetric review would have allowed optimised management and may have saved the life of Pamela's fetus.

Dr Feeney's discourteous conduct towards Josh Medhurst's parents (An avoidable tragedy) should not be tolerated. She may have had a reputation for bullying or being difficult. Josh's outcome may have been different if Dr Long had taken steps to have him reviewed earlier even if that meant incurring Dr Feeney's wrath.

INSIGHT

There are two aspects to this maxim. Both are major obstacles to safe medical practice.

The first is subjective. A reasonable medical practitioner should know the limits to his or her expertise or abilities. Proper introspection and performance evaluation should ensure that this occurs.

The second is objective and applies to cases where a professional colleague may be impaired, and a danger to patients. In the latter category, an effort should be made to communicate with the doctor in a compassionate way so that he or she is able to understand and accept the impairment. If these approaches to communicate are not met with positive behavioural changes, then more formal processes are indicated; such processes are in fact mandated under legislation. Several examples of these processes were discussed in the chapter about boundary violations.

The staff caring for Grace Campbell (Cerebral palsy) during her labour failed to seek advice and assistance from senior obstetric staff when there was incontrovertible evidence of fetal distress. Earlier consultation would likely have resulted in an emergency caesarean section, sparing Hayley from the effects of cerebral palsy. It is possible that the junior obstetric staff thought that they had the matter in hand, when they did not.

If Beryl Austin's overdose of heparin (Headache) had been discussed with specialists at the time the overdose was recognised, and not several hours later, steps could have been taken immediately to minimise the risk of intracranial bleeding. Specialists are known as specialists for a reason. They have specialised knowledge based on study and experience. Accessing their knowledge is as simple as a phone call. If this step had been taken in Beryl's case, she may well have avoided massive intracranial haemorrhage and premature death.

When performing the cholecystectomy on Liz Chadwick (Abdominal pain), Dr Briggs essentially got lost in the anatomy. He was not able to cannulate the cystic duct to perform an intraoperative cholangiogram, and his dissection was obviously inadequate because he did not identify the cystic duct and keep it from harm's way. Once he got into difficulty, he should have recognised that he was at the edge of his skill level, and asked for help from a specialist upper gastrointestinal tract surgeon.

Given Liz's condition immediately after the operation, Dr Briggs would have been better served by asking for a subspecialist to come in to advise about optimal management of his patient, rather than assuming he still had the expertise to deal with Liz's problems. If a surgeon with greater technical skill had been consulted earlier, then the outcome may have been better.

Professor Mulcahy (A mesh by any other name) did not advise Sue Massey that restrictions had been placed on his licence to practice, and falsely asserted that he would not use polypropylene mesh tapes in the proposed surgery for Sue. Sue's surgery was complicated by vaginal exposure of one of the tapes, for which she required additional surgery. She now has intractable pain, urinary incontinence, defaecatory obstruction and apareunia. Professor Mulcahy deceived Sue and she suffered for it.

Dr McIntyre did not disclose to Ahmad Abbas (Bladder cancer) that he had been banned from performing radical cystectomy neobladder surgery in the public hospital system because of unacceptable morbidity and mortality rates. Dr McIntyre offered and performed this surgery in a private hospital, with a poor outcome for Ahmad. If Dr McIntyre had disclosed his restrictions on practice, Ahmad would not have consented to surgery by Dr McIntyre and would have had the chance of a better outcome. And Dr McIntyre would have avoided another bad outcome.

Dr Franks, a recently appointed staff specialist obstetrician, had never performed the complex surgery required to safely deliver Simone Beall's second child (Placenta percreta). His registrar, Dr Dunn, was even less experienced, yet Dr Franks allowed Dr Dunn to be the lead surgeon. Baby Robert survived. Simone exsanguinated. If Dr Franks had consulted more experienced colleagues, a team of relevant specialists could have been assembled to plan and execute the surgery, with less risk than was the case with inexperienced operators who made numerous flawed surgical decisions.

Professionalism

While exercising care for a patient, a doctor should maintain a sense of professional detachment. Familiarity with a patient, including behaving as though the patient is a friend, can lead to blind spots in clinical judgment. At one end of the spectrum, such over-familiarity may lead to excessive investigation because a doctor might want to ensure that a friend is receiving the "very best treatment".

At the other end of the spectrum, over-familiarity could lead a doctor to assume that the presenting symptoms are a manifestation of some known personality trait such as hypochondriasis, and that it is thus unnecessary to investigate the matter more fully or at all.

Dr Fairweather assumed Steve Coates' weight loss (Unexplained weight loss) was due to his football training. If he was not familiar with the local footballer, he might have taken the presenting complaints more seriously.

Dr O'Toole must have realised that Mr Gladstone's protocol for rapid opioid detoxification fell outside the boundaries of usual care (A pharmacological nightmare). Dr O'Toole failed to exercise appropriate care in the prescription and administration of drugs without adequate clinical review beforehand.

Mr Gladstone failed to provide adequate supervision and resuscitation resources at his "clinic". Trudy Mawson lost her life as a result.

Boundary violations, of course, can be much more serious. Many psychiatric patients are vulnerable to boundary violations, the corollary being that the psychiatrist is also vulnerable to inappropriate relationships.

Dr Chung should have known that his conduct was going to put his patients and himself at risk of serious boundary violations (Post-traumatic stress disorder). He did nothing to protect himself let alone protect his patients. It was a major blind spot to safe psychiatric practice. The hospital at which he practised should also have put in place such things as therapy supervision to minimise the risk that serious boundary violations would occur. The absence of any safeguard resulted in Gabrielle being preyed upon by Dr Chung, and developing a severe aggravation of her post-traumatic stress disorder and depression.

Dr Banerjee (Ethical issues) was imprisoned for his abuse of Karima. Karima will bear her psychological scars for life. Doctors Black and Spalding were punished for taking advantage of their patients for their own gratification.

Dr Jackson declined to visit Sharon Monty (Asthma during pregnancy) on two occasions during the evening when nurses called her. Sharon was in her third trimester of pregnancy with twins. She had a long history of asthma and was in respiratory distress when the nurses called Dr Jackson. Dr Jackson left the nurses to manage Sharon overnight. When Dr Jackson eventually arrived to review Sharon the next day, Sharon was in extremis. The twins died in utero and Sharon died the following week. Dr Jackson had either failed to grasp the profound risk to Sharon and her unborn twins of asthma in advanced pregnancy, or she simply neglected her duty of care.

Dr Basri, who was a cardiologist, knew that Sally Kawolski (Ischaemic heart disease) had diabetes mellitus and ischaemic heart disease before he first saw her. Sally had been prescribed oral hypoglycaemic therapy, a statin and an angiotensin receptor blocker, but had not yet been prescribed antiplatelet therapy. For whatever reason, Dr Basri did not prescribe a platelet antagonist, and Sally had a heart attack the next year. If Dr Basri had discussed with Sally the risks and benefits of antiplatelet therapy, it is likely that Sally would have taken aspirin or clopidogrel, and may have avoided thrombotic coronary arterial occlusion. As it happened, the thrombosis was successfully treated with thrombolytic therapy.

When Sally returned to Dr Basri after her heart attack she was free of pain, and the only flow-limiting coronary stenosis was in a small branch of the right coronary artery. Without any functional testing to determine whether Sally had detectable reversible ischaemia, and without any discussion at a heart team meeting, Dr Basri proceeded to stent all three coronary arteries. Dr Basri received money for his interventions. Sally received stents which were not clinically indicated. She is now exposed to the risks of instent thrombosis and restenosis in all three coronary arteries, which would not have been the case without stenting.

Matthew Vella (Too many cooks) was attended by at least six different cardiologists, each of whom considered different aspects of his management. Nobody took responsibility for overall care. Matthew underwent coronary angiography which was not required. Dr Reddy did not question the indication for the procedure; he acquired unnecessary images and he failed to administer heparin. As a result of the procedure Matthew has permanent neurologic impairment.

Dr Feeney belittled the views of Julie Medhurst and Dr Sampson that Josh (An avoidable tragedy) had appendicitis. Dr Feeney refused to order an ultrasound or CT scan to exclude appendicitis. Expert care of Josh was delayed and he died as a result of his ruptured appendix. If Dr Feeney had been less belligerent, appropriate investigations would likely have been completed sooner than was the case, and there would likely have been time to save Josh's life.

LESSONS FOR DOCTORS AND OTHERS

There is no single explanation for the blind spots and roadblocks we have identified. Medical undergraduates receive their education from many sources. Some lecturers and clinical teachers are inspiring, and offer relevant messages clearly; some are not inspiring. Some areas of medicine may be covered comprehensively and effectively; others may not.

Although medical education may commence at university, that is just the beginning. Effective clinicians maintain their education and learning throughout their professional lives (including through participation in peer review, attendance at education sessions, keeping up-to-date with the literature and teaching others).

It is inevitable that junior doctors lack the experience of their senior colleagues. Accordingly it is necessary for systems of health care to provide adequate cognitive and physical support for junior doctors who manage potentially life-threatening situations (e.g. emergency department, birthing unit).

Medical graduates have competing priorities including work and family, income and expenditure, comprehensive care and numbers of patients to treat, and established protocols of care versus new and unproven technologies. Some doctors consult readily with others to obtain advice and direction; some practice in isolation. Some are affected by fatigue, mental illness, alcohol, drugs or sleep deprivation, and others may be distracted by personal and financial issues.

Some doctors work in an environment where it is easy to confer informally with others in a nonthreatening way; some work in a multidoctor practice but have little face-to-face interaction with colleagues; and others choose to work solo, and may take few holidays, and may spend little time on continuing education. Most medical practitioners maintain effective continuing education and peer review (as they are required to do); others do not.

Basic knowledge is essential. It is sometimes challenging to recognise what you do not know. Nevertheless, failure of cognition may be overcome to some extent by paying careful attention to the lessons enumerated below.

Lessons for Doctors

The lessons which flow from the cases we have presented are simple, and can be employed by all medical practitioners. Here they are:

1. History

It is vital to spend sufficient time to elicit the relevant history. This may require an interpreter, and it may require more than one consultation.

It is important to recognise potential impediments to history taking, including age, gender, faith, ethnicity, body habitus, mental health, intoxication and social traits. It may be necessary for the practitioner to vary his or her usual manner of history taking to suit different patients and different circumstances to avoid missing important information. It may be necessary to continue history taking after the patient has sobered-up or had a wash.

2. Examination

The relevant part or parts should be adequately exposed and examined systematically. Shortcuts should be avoided. Reexamination on different days may be required to observe changes. The same comments about impediments to history taking apply to physical examination.

3. Diagnosis

Always consider potentially serious diagnoses before opting for a benign diagnosis with no differentials, and always consider and exclude an organic cause for psychiatric symptoms.

Be prepared to revise an initial diagnosis and consider new differentials if the clinical course is inconsistent with the initial diagnosis.

Remember that common things occur commonly.

4. Tests

If in doubt about the significance of a result, consult with an experienced colleague. This is especially important when doctors are inexperienced in managing a particular condition (whether soon after graduation or later in practising life). The same principle applies to interpretation of the literature in respect of new therapies or investigative modalities.

Always check that test results, and opinions of consultants, are received and reviewed appropriately.

5. Communication

Take the necessary time to communicate with the patient and family. Record details of clinical encounters adequately. Review tests and pass on the results to relevant parties in a timely manner.

This communication time is in addition to the time taken to elicit the history. Remember that some patients may not be able to assimilate complex sets of information and strategies at one sitting, and may require multiple encounters in order to understand issues and make informed decisions.

6. Knowledge

In addition to mandatory requirements for continuing education, ensure that you have adequate peer review, and avoid unnecessary shortcuts in clinical practice. Ensure that current guidelines for investigation and treatment are reviewed and implemented.

7. Advocate

Always be an unbiased advocate for your patient when considering therapeutic options.

It is correct to consider new management techniques, but it remains vital to offer a balanced view to patients and their families when comparing the value and suitability of new techniques with established ones.

8. Fallibility

Always be prepared to admit experiencing difficulty with a procedure, at the time of the difficulty. Experienced colleagues are usually available to offer advice by phone or otherwise, or physical assistance if necessary. It is never sensible to pretend that a difficulty or complication has not occurred.

9. Bias

If you are invited to serve as an expert witness, it is your responsibility to provide honest and unbiased opinions to assist the court. It is not appropriate, and not helpful to anyone, to act as a hired-gun on behalf of one side or another.

10. Risk

These lessons cannot guarantee avoidance of all errors, but attention to these lessons will help to minimise the risk of inadvertently causing harm to a patient or to one's reputation.

Lessons for Others

The lessons above do not apply to doctors in isolation from society otherwise.

Governments

Governments at all levels have a responsibility to establish and maintain systems to facilitate safe and cost-effective health care. As medical practices evolve, in the context of society generally, the character of such systems must be adapted to take account of evolving medical practices (e.g. subspecialisation, telemedicine, electronic records). This means appropriate resource allocation is required (adjusted from time to time) to provide optimal care for patients and appropriate remuneration for health workers, including doctors.

The legal framework to deal with medical litigation should ideally provide equitable compensation for injured patients without unnecessary legal and court costs.

The promulgation of diagnostic and treatment guidelines needs to be considered carefully. Guidelines are important aids to medical practitioners, but they should not be followed blindly. Guidelines should not prevent the application of individualised clinical judgment.

Medical schools

Medical educators need to revise their curricula from time to time to adjust to changing medical knowledge. In the process of making changes to the content of medical education, care must be taken to emphasise the keystone role of basic clinical principles in the practice of medicine, and not to favour exposure to niche subspecialties at the expense of adequate teaching of basic clinical principles.

The best medical educators will ensure that their students develop systems of clinical behaviour that will facilitate life-long learning and professional development.

Credentialling bodies

Credentialling and regulatory bodies need to provide a framework to ensure that high standards of medical practice are encouraged, without unnecessary red tape.

Practitioner representatives

Professional medical colleges and representative groups must advise government, credentialling bodies, medical schools and hospital administrators of ways by which systems may be improved to ensure patient safety and doctor satisfaction.

Hospitals

Hospital administrators need to balance the requirements of safe patient care against budgetary constraints. Junior doctors require supervision and support. Senior doctors require review of their practices to ensure that standards are maintained. All practitioners should be encouraged to participate in peer review and continuing education. Systems of communication should enable junior staff to negotiate the authority gradient to optimise patient care.

Patients

Patients and their families are entitled to expect thoughtful and compassionate care from their doctors. Patients and their families should be made comfortable to ask questions about medical care options and costs. Those questions should be answered honestly and without bias.

Patients should be aware that medical blind spots and roadblocks exist, and be prepared at any time to request additional opinions if they are concerned about the quality of their care.

FURTHER READING

Clinical Negligence (Powers and Barton: Bloomsbury Professional) provides information about legal and medical aspects of clinical negligence in England.

The Australian Medico-Legal Handbook (Kerridge, Stewart and Parker: Elsevier) addresses a broad range of legal and ethical issues associated with medical practice.

Complications (Gawande: Profile Books) describes a range of surgical misadventures.

The reader is encouraged to refer to specialty literature for additional information about the various conditions discussed.

ABBREVIATIONS

AD	anno domini
AF	atrial fibrillation
AHPRA	Australian Health Practitioner Regulation Agency
APGAR	neonatal scoring system including appearance, pulse, grimace, activity and respiration
APTT	activated partial thromboplastin time, to assess anticoagulation
ARTG	Australian Register of Therapeutic Goods
BC	before Christ
BMI	boy mass index kg/m^2
c	circa (approximate year)
CCF	congestive cardiac failure
CPR	cardiorespiratory resuscitation
CRP	C-reactive protein
CT	computed tomogram
DVT	deep vein thrombosis
ECG	electrocardiogram (usually 12-lead)
ENT	ear, nose and throat
ERCP	endoscopic retrograde cholangiopancreatogram
ESR	erythrocyte sedimentation rate
et seq.	and what follows
FDA	Food and Drug Administration (US)
FRACGP	Fellow of The Royal Australian College of General Practitioners
HCCC	Health Care Complaints Commission
HCG	human chorionic gonadotropin
HPCA	Health Professional Councils Authority
HPV	human papilloma virus
INT	intermediate artery
LFTs	liver function tests
LIMA	left internal mammary artery
LMCA	left main coronary artery
LRA	left radial artery
MFM	maternal fetal medicine
MSSA	methicillin-sensitive Staphylococcus aureus
MRA	magnetic resonance angiography
MRI	magnetic resonance imaging
NASH	nonalcoholic steatohepatitis
NCAT	NSW Civil and Administrative Tribunal
PDA	posterior descending artery

PEG	percutaneous endoscopic gastrostomy
PFO	patent foramen ovale
PICU	paediatric intensive care unit
PLCX	posterolateral circumflex artery
POP	pelvic organ prolapse
RANZCOG	Royal Australian and New Zealand College of Obstetricians and Gynaecologists
RCA	right coronary artery
RIMA	right internal mammary artery
SAH	subarachnoid haemorrhage
SCC	squamous cell carcinoma
STEMI	ST elevation myocardial infarction
SUI	stress urinary incontinence
TCC	transitional cell carcinoma
tds	three times daily
TFS	tissue fixation system
UVB	ultraviolet B

INDEX

Page numbers followed by "*t*" indicate tables.

D

E

F

P

S